Ethics for Health Professionals

Carla Caldwell Stanford, PhD, CFLE

Valerie J. Connor, MA, CCC-SLP

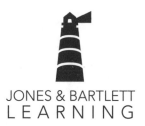

JONES & BARTLETT
LEARNING

World Headquarters
Jones & Bartlett Learning
5 Wall Street
Burlington, MA 01803
978-443-5000
info@jblearning.com
www.jblearning.com

Jones & Bartlett Learning books and products are available through most bookstores and online booksellers. To contact Jones & Bartlett Learning directly, call 800-832-0034, fax 978-443-8000, or visit our website, www.jblearning.com.

Substantial discounts on bulk quantities of Jones & Bartlett Learning publications are available to corporations, professional associations, and other qualified organizations. For details and specific discount information, contact the special sales department at Jones & Bartlett Learning via the above contact information or send an email to specialsales@jblearning.com.

Ethics for Health Professionals is an independent publication and has not been authorized, sponsored, or otherwise approved by the owners of the trademarks or service marks referenced in this product.

Some images in this book feature models. These models do not necessarily endorse, represent, or participate in the activities represented in the images.

The authors, editor, and publisher have made every effort to provide accurate information. However, they are not responsible for errors, omissions, or for any outcomes related to the use of the contents of this book and take no responsibility for the use of the products and procedures described. Treatments and side effects described in this book may not be applicable to all people; likewise, some people may require a dose or experience a side effect that is not described herein. Drugs and medical devices are discussed that may have limited availability controlled by the Food and Drug Administration (FDA) for use only in a research study or clinical trial. Research, clinical practice, and government regulations often change the accepted standard in this field. When consideration is being given to use of any drug in the clinical setting, the health care provider or reader is responsible for determining FDA status of the drug, reading the package insert, and reviewing prescribing information for the most up-to-date recommendations on dose, precautions, and contraindications, and determining the appropriate usage for the product. This is especially important in the case of drugs that are new or seldom used.

Production Credits

Publisher: William Brottmiller
Acquisitions Editor: Katey Birtcher
Associate Editor: Teresa Reilly
Associate Production Editor: Jill Morton
Marketing Manager: Grace Richards
Manufacturing and Inventory Control
  Supervisor: Amy Bacus
Composition: Cenveo Publisher Services

Cover Design: Scott Moden
Rights & Photo Research Assistant:
  Miranda Rivers
Cover Image: Scales, © allegro/ShutterStock, Inc.;
  Medical caduceus,
  © Maximus256/ShutterStock, Inc.
Printing and Binding: Edwards Brothers Malloy
Cover Printing: Edwards Brothers Malloy

To order this product, use ISBN: 978-1-4496-8960-5

Library of Congress Cataloging-in-Publication Data
Stanford, Carla Caldwell, 1959-
  Ethics for health professionals / by Carla Caldwell Stanford and Valerie J. Connor.
     p. ; cm.
  Includes bibliographical references and index.
  ISBN 978-1-4496-7832-6 — ISBN 1-4496-7832-7
  I. Connor, Valerie J. II. Title.
  [DNLM: 1. Ethics, Clinical. 2. Professional-Patient Relations—ethics. WB 60]

  174.2—dc23
                        2012023893

6048

Printed in the United States of America

Contents

Foreword

This world, for many, presents a hungry quest to "get ahead," and ethics is not always the first consideration in any given scenario. Lines once starkly black have faded to gray. Why do you suppose that is? Confronted with ethical uncertainty, it has become more important than ever to embrace a set of values and attitudes. Knowing yourself includes knowing these values. In what do you believe? Where do you draw lines when it comes to controversial matters? Throughout this text, you should reflect on your own set of beliefs and values.

The healthcare professional will daily be faced with decision-making tasks, both on the job and off. Today's healthcare industry is overshadowed, for some, by the threat of being sued. Consequently, tasks are sometimes met with reserve and what-ifs. Throughout this text, you will read about ethical situations. Combining your own personal values system and new information in this text, you should consider all angles and come to conclusions through reasoning skills.

As you begin this text, think about what you currently know about ethics. Keep an open mind about new information to which you will be introduced so that you can use all available information to arrive at a conclusion. When you come to the end of the text, gauge your growth in this field by comparing your new knowledge of ethics to your earlier knowledge base, and explore your opinions and feelings about healthcare ethics.

Good luck as you begin this learning journey, and best wishes to you in your upcoming career in health care!

Acknowledgments

In a world of "me, me, me," it is with warmth that I remember the people who accept me as I am and to whom I owe my own ethical standards: my husband Allen; my three sons Will, Hunter, and Ryne; my daughters-in-law Mary Frances and Lauren; and my precious granddaughter Anna Lyn. You are the heart of all that I am, and I love you all very much. My faith is the foundation for my ethical beliefs, steeped heavily in childhood lessons by my parents.

Thanks to all who have shown support throughout this writing process and who offered encouragement and help, including those who reviewed and provided quotes and resource materials. A textbook, I have found firsthand, is the writing of one or more (two in this case), but the collaboration of many. My hope is that students who read it will be enriched by ethical information that will last a lifetime. Students are dear to my heart, and I admire anyone for bettering themselves through higher education. Knowledge truly is power.

Finally, I want to acknowledge my colleague and coauthor, Valerie Connor, who is not only kind, patient, and reliable, but also knowledgeable in the field of ethics within the healthcare industry. I can think of no one with whom I would have rather taken this journey. Thanks, Val!

—Carla Caldwell Stanford

I would like to thank my wonderful husband, Martin, who provided encouragement and multiple hours of proofreading! A big thank you to our two children, Quinn and Savannah, who never run out of love and words of support. I love all of you very much!

There have been many people in my life who have provided me with opportunities as a speech therapist and an educator. The writing process has enriched my knowledge of the field of healthcare ethics, and I hope this textbook will inspire students to keep learning.

Finally, a big thank you to Carla Stanford, who convinced me that I could coauthor a textbook, provided countless hours of guidance and encouraging e-mails, and never doubted our success. You are the best!

—Valerie J. Connor

Reviewers

Cheryl L. DiLanzo, MS, RT (R)
Clinical Coordinator
Montgomery County Community College
Blue Bell, PA

Elgloria A. Harrison, MS, RRT, NPS, AE-C
Associate Professor
Chair, Nursing and Health Professions
University of the District of Columbia
Washington, DC

Jim Hinojosa, PhD, OT, BCP, FAOTA
Professor
Steinhardt School of Culture, Education, and Human Development
New York University
New York, NY

Kathleen O. Kienstra, MAT, RT (R)(T)
Program Director, Radiation Therapy
Saint Louis University
St. Louis, MO

Gerard Magill, PhD
Vernon F. Gallagher Chair and Professor of Healthcare Ethics
Center for Healthcare Ethics
Duquesne University, Pittsburgh
Pittsburgh, PA

About the Authors

Carla Caldwell Stanford holds two master's degrees and a PhD. She has taught a medical law and bioethics course at the undergraduate college level for five years. The motivating factor for writing a textbook was to simplify ethics and laws concerning the healthcare professional in ways that would be both appealing and easily understood by the student.

Valerie J. Connor has a master's degree in speech pathology. She has practiced in school and long-term care settings. Currently, she teaches at both the undergraduate and graduate level with a focus on the legal and ethical aspects of health care. She hopes that students will have a better understanding of the laws and ethical issues surrounding health care after reading this text.

Chapter 1

An Overview of Ethics

Even the most rational approach to ethics is defenseless if there isn't the will to do what is right.

—Alexander Solzhenitsyn, Russian novelist and Nobel Prize winner

KEY TERMS

Applied ethics	Meta-ethics
Consequence	Normative ethics
Consequential approach	Personal values system
Deontology	Rights-based ethics
Dilemma	Three-Step Ethical
Duty-based ethics	Decision-Making Model
Ethics	Utilitarian-based ethics
Inductive reasoning	Virtue-based ethics

AN OVERVIEW OF ETHICS

When you hear the word *ethics*, what comes to mind? For many people, ethics means right versus wrong. However, our definition should not stop there. **Ethics** is a branch of philosophy concerning moral considerations, but how each person reaches conclusions about those considerations is subjective, meaning the process varies from person to person.

To help illustrate the subjectivity of ethics, let's take a look at an industry unrelated to health care: fashion. Fashion trends run in cycles, largely influenced by political conditions, economics, and popular fads. What one person views as fashionable another might view as hideous, pretentious, or boring. Though great designers such as Versace and Givenchy set trends, it is up to the individual to decide what he or she finds attractive. The 1970s brought us bell-bottoms and platform shoes, and while many followed the trend and sales on these clothing items skyrocketed during this time, there were still many people who did not like the appearance of bell-bottoms and platform shoes and did not purchase them. Those who wore these items might look back and ask, "What was I thinking?"

So it is with ethics: The individual dictates what is "right" or "wrong" within the personal realm. Why, then, are there so many views on any one given topic? It is because each individual possesses a unique set of experiences and influences that guide his or her personal values system. A **personal values system** is a set of beliefs held by an individual. These beliefs may overlap with other factors. Influences on a person's values system could include any of the following:

- Religion
- Socioeconomic conditions
- Family and friends
- Geographic location
- Cultural and heritage traditions

The health care professional must acquire a very specific set of skills that coincides with his or her field of expertise. For example, the medical assistant must learn to properly sterilize medical instruments. Along with that and other job skills, the medical assistant must learn the art of caring for patients, including legal and ethical considerations (**Figure 1-1**).

If you subscribe to the notion that humans have an "inner voice" (some call this a conscience), you might believe this voice to be ethically sound. Ethics is a morally based field, meaning that this branch of philosophy corresponds with human morals. It is important, however, to remember that a person's conscience and ethics are distinctly different. Ethics are guided by society and are a series of systematic beliefs, while the conscience refers to thoughts about one's beliefs and actions. Both the conscience and ethics have been around since the beginning of human history.

Consider the caveman who lived by sheer survival device yet still congregated into groups with others of similar interests. There is evidence that humans of this era shunned those who did not agree with their codes of conduct, even expelling them from the group. Based on this, we can feel confident that their values systems, based

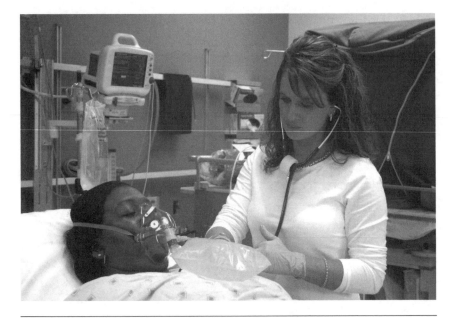

Figure 1-1 A healthcare professional with a patient.

on ethics, guided their beliefs and actions. This, then, would support the belief that ethics, on some level, is "built into" our very being (intrinsic). How each of us interprets each ethical situation, though, varies greatly.

Now that you have some basic knowledge about ethics, let's look at some early influences on the field.

EARLY INFLUENCES ON THE FIELD OF ETHICS

Many great thinkers have contributed to the field of ethics. For this discussion we will focus on two philosophers: Socrates and Confucius. Though many would regard Socrates (ancient Greek philosopher) as the Father of Ethics, others might proclaim that Confucius and his teachings set the foundation for organized thinking about ethics. You be the judge. Here, we will discuss the significant contributions of each.

For Your Consideration

Confucius and Socrates lived and taught before Plato and Aristotle. In fact, Plato was a student of Socrates. Aristotle was a student of Plato. Do some Web surfing (on reliable sites) and find others who followed these philosophers. What did they contribute, and what do these contributions mean to the healthcare professional?

Confucius

Confucius (born with the name Kong) was born in 552 BC in Lu, China (**Figure 1-2**). During his life, the slave system in the East was on the brink of collapse. As with any of us, he was heavily influenced

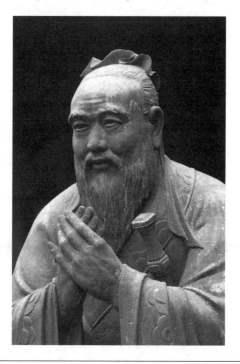

Figure 1-2 Statue of Confucius at Confucian Temple in Shanghai, China.

by his location and by the political conditions of the region. In fact, he was so dedicated that he divorced his wife to fully devote himself to his studies. Soon after his divorce, his mother died. This event marked another sad passage in his life—one that would influence many others. At that time (around 529 BC), the practice of memorializing the remains of the deceased had practically been discontinued by Easterners. Confucius could not see overlooking such a tribute, so he held a solemn service honoring his beloved mother. Afterward, others began to follow his lead and held services for their dead loved ones. This perhaps has influenced such traditions of today.

Confucius was heartbroken and confined himself to seclusion for 3 years, at which time he fully devoted himself to study and reflection. When he emerged from isolation, he began teaching what he had learned. His followers were not the typical students of the time, but men who were considered pillars of the community and wielded great influence. Confucius also traveled throughout his country but was never given the respect as in his home area. In fact, not only was he shunned, he was imprisoned and almost starved to death.

Returning to his homeland penniless and disheartened, he poured himself into writing.

During his lifetime, he was not appreciated for his wisdom. His writings began the Ju (or Confucianism) movement but were not recognized as praiseworthy until after his death in 479 BC.

Notable Confucius quotes (BrainyQuote, 2012a):
- Faced with what is right, to leave it undone shows a lack of courage.
- I hear and I forget. I see and I remember. I do and I understand.
- Choose a job you love and you will never have to work a day in your life.
- Our greatest glory is not in never falling, but in rising every time we fall.
- The superior man thinks always of virtue; the common man thinks of comfort.

Socrates

Socrates, known by many as the Father of Democracy, was born in Athens, Greece, in 470 BC (**Figure 1-3**). His father was a stonecutter/sculptor, and his mother was a midwife. Socrates often compared the study of philosophy to his parents' professions, particularly his mother's. He even called himself "a midwife of ideas." In his younger life, he was a Greek soldier, which is perhaps the opposite of what you might expect from a philosopher whom we associate with peace and resolution.

He seldom stayed home, though he had a wife and three children; according to some, he even took a second wife, which was permitted by a polygamy law of the time. Instead, on any given day, he could be found near the court square teaching. He was seen as arrogant by some because he was so blunt. In fact, his blunt depiction of local leaders soon made Socrates a target of public officials. He once said

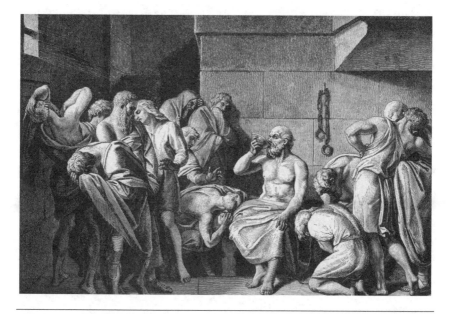

Figure 1-3 Socrates drinking the Conium. Engraved by unknown engraver and published in *Pictorial History of the World's Great Nations, United States, 1882.*

that only philosophers should govern, because only they were fit for the job. Ironically, he himself never held office.

Socrates was accused of corrupting the young minds of students and of impiety (questioning the existence of the gods and not worshiping gods of the state). He denied these charges but was still condemned to death by a jury of over 500. He was sentenced to death by drinking hemlock, a poison (Pima County, Arizona, n.d.).

Socrates' teachings centered on **inductive reasoning**, which is critical thinking that moves from specific details to generalities. For example, a medical assistant might observe that Mrs. Studdard always seems to have headaches when she comes into the ABC Clinic. After many tests, it is learned that Mrs. Studdard has high blood pressure. When given medication for this condition, her headaches disappear. Thus, it could be induced that high blood pressure causes headaches. From this induction, a person could prove or disprove this theory based on more observations. Of course, we know that high blood pressure does not always cause headaches, but it certainly could be generalized to many patients—just not all patients.

Teaching by asking questions, as Socrates often did, has become known as the Socratic method of teaching. Instead of simply lecturing to his students, Socrates would ask questions that would cause them to reflect in a deeper, more meaningful way. While elaborating on what the student might say or ask, Socrates would encourage open discussion and sorting of the subject matter. Even today, many educators use this *Socratic method* in teaching.

Notable Socrates quotes (BrainyQuote, 2012b):
- The only true wisdom is in knowing you know nothing.
- He is a man of courage who does not run away, but remains at his post and fights against the enemy.
- Let him that would move the world first move himself.
- The unexamined life is not worth living.
- The way to gain a good reputation is to endeavor to be what you desire to appear.

MAJOR AREAS OF ETHICAL PHILOSOPHY

How you arrive at your own beliefs and attitudes is influenced by your life experiences, you education, and those around you (family, friends, coworkers, teachers, neighbors, and others). For example, those living in the "Bible Belt" of the southeastern United States might find that geographic location, culture/heritage, and religion all intersect to form their perspectives on such issues as abortion, whatever those perspectives might be. A person's perspective on these issues might be different in another part of the country. The saying that "No man is an island" holds true, as no person can ever come to conclusions without external influence, whatever that influence may be.

Can you think of specific examples of your viewpoint(s) of issues that might have been externally influenced? While reading this text, you should learn to survey your own feelings and opinions on ethically based topics. By becoming more aware of your own values system, you will be more equipped to confront and cope with ethical scenarios.

Ethics is a complex subject divided into distinct areas. Experts often propose different approaches to these areas. We will only introduce the basic approaches in this text. The following outline might help you understand their connection:

I. Meta-ethics
II. Normative ethics
   A. Virtue-based
   B. Consequential approach
      1. Utilitarianism
   C. Duty-based (also known as rights-based ethics or deontology)
III. Applied ethics

Do not confuse the major areas of study (i.e., meta-ethics, normative ethics, and applied ethics) with the approaches to those areas (i.e., virtue-based, duty-based, and consequential approach, which includes utilitarianism) (Fieser, 2003). The *areas* of ethical study define the types of ethical philosophy, while the *approaches* to ethical study

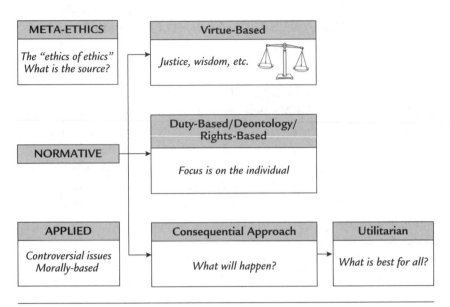

Figure 1-4 Making sense of the areas of ethics.

present ways to arrive at decisions about ethical dilemmas. In other words, dilemmas fall within the three major areas of study, and the approaches are simply ways of applying or using that area of study (**Figure 1-4**).

Major Area 1: Meta-Ethics

To understand **meta-ethics**, we need only to understand the nature of ethics and the source. Perhaps we could maintain that it is the *ethics of ethics*, since the word *meta* (from the Greek) means "beyond" and in some interpretations "after." This definition would suggest that meta-ethics is a more intensive examination of ethics. Interestingly enough, the very fact that you are reading this would assume that you are engaged in the study of meta-ethics since you are considering its meaning. In meta-ethics, you do not decide right from wrong; rather you decide what the terms "right" and "wrong" really mean. Meta-ethics is more intense and often abstract in nature. Instead of arriving at a conclusion about an ethical dilemma, using meta-ethics as a basis, you instead investigate deeper thoughts such as:

- What exactly constitutes "good" or "bad"?
- Is morality the same for everyone, or is it determined on a case-by-case basis?
- From where do morals originate?
- Is there only one answer to any given ethical dilemma?

Major Area 2: Normative Ethics

Normative ethics involves those standards by which right and wrong are determined within a society. For example, the Golden Rule, "Do unto others as you would have them do unto you," is normative. You make decisions based on what you know to be appropriate. Applying this way of thinking, you do not want others to steal from you, so you should not steal from others.

In normative ethics, it is assumed that there is only one fundamental measurement for any given behavior or attitude, whether it is a single principle or a set of principles. Within the normative ethics, there are three strategies: (1) virtue-based, (2) consequential, and (3) duty-based.

Approach 1: Virtue-Based Ethics

The foundation of the first approach, **virtue-based ethics**, is the individual's choice of values (virtues), with decisions and actions being based on the corresponding values systems. Virtue-based ethics concern decisions that encourage the most admirable of virtues within a person's character. Practicing these virtues every day will help them become habit. This strategy has its roots in Western civilization, stemming from the teaching of Plato (student of Socrates). He saw four main traits (later to be called the *cardinal virtues*) as particularly important: wisdom, courage, temperance, and justice. What other virtues can you list? (Note: Do not get virtues and priorities confused. For example, family, education, and success are priorities, not virtues. They would fall into duty-based ethics, discussed later. Other virtues could include honesty and perseverance.)

Approach 2: The Consequential Approach

In the second approach, the **consequential approach**, issues are judged as intrinsically (from within) good or bad, with the decision being based on what will bring about the best balance of good outcomes over bad. It is, then, logical that what is good and bad might be viewed differently depending on the person judging. The easy way to relate the consequential approach is to consider its root word, **consequence**, which refers to the result of an action. There are many types of consequential approaches; we will only discuss the most widely known, utilitarianism.

Utilitarianism

The utilitarian view is perhaps the most renowned type of consequential ethics, coming about in the 1700s. **Utilitarian-based ethics** suggests that the decision to ethical dilemmas should be based on the choice that is best for the majority. In this approach, you are called upon to be unbiased and not consider your own interests ahead of others'. Legal systems are quite often utilitarian, as those involved in them (attorneys, judges, juries, etc.) primarily consider the safety of and fairness to society. As stated by Mack (2004):

> While it is generally agreed that sensible moral norms will promote the interest of individuals and of society, utilitarians go one step further than that. They take the view that the only rational basis for our compliance with various moral norms is the benefit this provides for us and for society as a whole.

Case Study: Utilitarianism

Imagine you are a hospital administrator. You currently are trying to recruit Dr. Carlisle Ferrerro, a world-renowned physician/researcher in the field of sudden infant death syndrome (SIDS), to come practice and do ground-breaking research at your hospital.

Funding his project and paying him what he requires would mean sacrificing a great portion of your benevolent funds, which support the in-house Free Clinic to those who cannot afford health care.

The work of Dr. Ferrerro is indisputably important in saving lives, but the Free Clinic serves hundreds of patients who might not otherwise be able to receive health care. Do you lessen the services of the Free Clinic (including laying off employees) to hire Dr. Ferrerro, or do you decide to keep the Free Clinic open and not hire Dr. Ferrerro?

It would seem that the Ferrerro decision lies in the "here and now," which is the existing clinic, versus the future factor, which is Dr. Ferrerro's research and the lives it will save. If you are using the utilitarian approach in this case, you will look at the benefits on each side of the dilemma and choose the one that serves the most people. This would call for unbiased calculations of the facts and arrive at numbers to support the solution that would help the most people, based on ethical standards. How do you think you would act in this instance?

Approach 3: Duty-Based Ethics, Also Known as Deontology

You just read about good versus bad in the consequential approach and how it focuses on what is best for the majority. Let us now examine the third and final approach within normative ethics—the individual as the center of attention. **Duty-based ethics**, also known as **deontology** or **rights-based ethics**, maintains that certain life obligations should be of primary focus in a person's everyday life (Tooley, n.d.). Those obligations should take priority over other considerations. In deontological-based ethics, the individual's rights are most important, so what is best for the individual cannot be precluded by what is best for the *greater good.* Deontologists believe that it is wrong to violate individual rights for the sake of a possible better situation for more people. When you think of individual rights, such terms as religion, speech, and safety probably come to mind.

Case Study: Deontology

In the hypothetical country of Bernard, there is a great wave of a new strain of influenza B (one that only affects humans). Though Bernardian medical professionals have made every effort to treat those affected, the Thunder Flu, as it is called, has already killed 400 people, with another 2,400 infected and in critical condition. The quarantine of patients to the main hospital in the region has not helped, so government officials gather to decide what to do, with the advice of the medical community. If patients are not soon moved or healed, the entire Bernardian population could be destroyed.

Off the coast of Bernard is Aquarian Island, which is also part of the country. There are no modern conveniences such as electricity or modern communication on Aquarian. The island is also overrun by snakes and is dense in forests. At the insistence of the majority of Bernardian officials, it was decided that all infected with Thunder Flu must be evacuated immediately to Aquarian. These people will have no electricity and no communication outlets, and will not be allowed to communicate with anyone not on the island. No doctors will be sent, and only a limited supply of food, water, and basic provisions will be distributed. It is expected that the people will eventually die out (most likely within a month). The orders are instantly carried out and the infected patients are exiled to Aquarian despite protests from the patients themselves and others in the country.

This may seem to be an extreme example, but it drives home the fact that those who contracted Thunder Flu were stripped of all rights and left to die. According to deontology, what would be the argument for not moving the Thunder Flu patients to Aquarian?

In deontology, it is believed that it is wrong and immoral to assume that one person is more deserving of something than someone else is. Unlike with the consequential approach and the utilitarian approaches, the *greater good* is not considered because it weakens the rights of the individual.

Major Area 3: Applied Ethics

Applied ethics is a major area of ethics that calls for the investigation of any given debate over a morally based issue. There are two aspects of an applied ethical dilemma: (1) it is an issue that is controversial (meaning, there are more than one viewpoint on the issue) and (2) it is clearly classified as a moral issue. Examples of this would include abortion, euthanasia, and stem cell research. Not included in applied ethics are traffic laws, political elections, and Homeland Security because these three and many others do not address controversial, morally based ethics for the most part. As Fieser states, a drive-by shooting would not involve applied ethics because most would agree it is immoral. However, gun control (which is a broader issue) would involve applied ethics (Fieser, 2003).

In applied ethics it would seem that the answer is clear on a given matter. Let's look at euthanasia as an example. If the patient is in intolerable pain and has stated that he does not want to be "kept alive by machines," it would seem that euthanasia is the obvious answer. But what if that patient only stated verbally his wishes (nothing in writing) and the family does not want to end his life? It is then that the issue becomes controversial and requires deep reflection as to what is most appropriate in this situation. Controversy only occurs when there is more than one viewpoint on an issue.

ETHICAL DECISION MAKING

Whether it be choosing to send sick people to an island, as the Bernard case study considered, or to cross the street, you make decisions (both major and minor) many times throughout the day. If you think about it, the entire healthcare profession and the services rendered are based on decisions, such as:

- What are the patient's symptoms?
- What is the best course of treatment?

- Does the medication given, if any, have side effects that might be harmful to the patient?
- Is hospitalization or home health services more appropriate?
- Should the injection be given in the arm or in the hip?

The list could go on and on. That is why the consummate health-care professional should be equipped with the latest knowledge of any given disease and the skill sets to provide the best care for the patient. *Knowledge combined with skills plus a caring attitude make for the best patient care possible.* Decision making is important to the patient because it could be a matter of life and death; at the very least, it is a matter of health.

The Three-Step Ethical Decision-Making Model

There is no right way to do a wrong thing.

—From *The Power of Ethical Management* by Blanchard and Peale

Some decisions, like body movements, are made automatically (or involuntarily), while other decisions must be contemplated. In the field of health care, you will be faced with a great many important ethical dilemmas that require contemplation. A **dilemma** is a crisis or situation in which a decision is required in order for change or improvement to occur. When decision time comes, you might consider using the **Three-Step Ethical Decision-Making Model** as presented by Kenneth Blanchard and Norman Vincent Peale in their book *The Power of Ethical Management* **(Figure 1-5)**. This model was created to help individuals make decisions at work, but it can help you make decisions on any ethical dilemma. Commit it to memory and use it when you need to make a difficult decision:

1. Is it legal?
2. Is it balanced?
3. How does it make me feel?

Is It Legal?

Laws are based on what is believed to be fair and just. Laws serve as guides you must follow to be a law-abiding citizen. In making

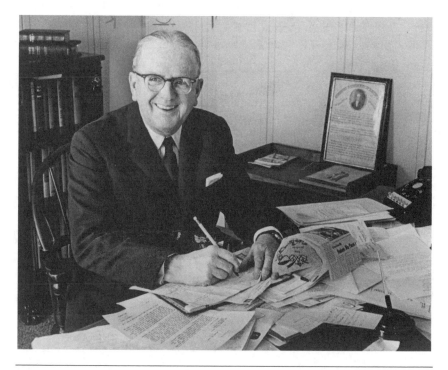

Figure 1-5 Norman Vincent Peale.

any moral decision, it can be presupposed that if something is not legal, it is not ethical. Therefore, if you ask yourself, "Is it legal?" and the answer is "no," there is no need to go further in the Three-Step Model.

Is It Balanced?

Balance, as Socrates believed, is important to the well-rounded individual. "All work and no play makes Jack a dull boy" is still a true statement. If something seems extreme to you, it is most likely not balanced. Being dedicated to a sport is commendable, but doing so in an extreme manner is out of balance. For example, an athlete who practices 8 hours a day in the off-season and still does not get the results he or she desires might resort to steroids. This is, of course, not only illegal, but out of balance.

How Does It Make Me Feel?

How *you* feel is an all-essential factor in decision making, so your feelings should not be ignored. How you feel is most likely a product of your conscious and subconscious beliefs about any given matter. Have you ever done something then felt so guilty it almost made you sick? This is just one example of how your feelings guide you mentally, and as in this case, physically.

Trivia Quest

Dr. Norman Vincent Peale, coauthor of *The Power of Ethical Management*, was one of the greatest spiritual leaders of his time. He was author of more than 40 books and personal advisor to two American presidents (Eisenhower and Nixon). Still widely read today, perhaps his most memorable writing was *The Power of Positive Thinking* (1952).

PUTTING IT ALL TOGETHER

The pioneers of ethical thinking, such as Socrates and Confucius, laid a firm foundation on which to build our own personal values system. Those who followed them would further investigate and expand on their work. Consider the three major areas of ethics studies: meta-ethics, normative ethics, and applied ethics. To which area do you most relate? The truth is, if we are balanced in our thinking (as the Three-Step Model would encourage), we would find that we will use all three areas from time to time.

Decision making, whether conscious or unconscious, is the task of every human. However, decision making in health care involves intentional reflection. The decisions that healthcare professionals make on a daily basis are largely matters that affect people's well-being and could be matters of life and death. The healthcare professional deals with heavy decisions, not to be taken lightly. Knowing your own values will help you arrive at a logical and practical conclusion that will be the most appropriate choice. Practice and experience will enhance your decision-making skills.

CHAPTER CHECKUP

Matching

Identify each statement with one of the following major areas of ethics study:

A. Meta-ethics
B. Normative ethics
C. Applied ethics

1. _____ Is guided by society.
2. _____ Involves highly controversial issues.
3. _____ The ethics of ethics.
4. _____ Involves deep reflection.
5. _____ Three subsets under this area are duty-based, virtue-based, and consequential.
6. _____ Asks, "What is the source?"
7. _____ Utilitarianism is the most widely known approach to this area.
8. _____ The Golden Rule is an example of this.

Identify each statement with one of the following people:

A. Socrates
B. Confucius

1. _____ Isolated himself to fully focus on his studies
2. _____ Was highly regarded for his wisdom only after his death
3. _____ Was sentenced to death by drinking hemlock (poison)
4. _____ Taught in the court square
5. _____ Lived in Athens, Greece
6. _____ Lived in Lu, China
7. _____ Died penniless
8. _____ Father of Democracy

Fill-in-the-Blank

1. _____ is a branch of philosophy concerning moral considerations.
2. Name three factors that can influence a person's values system:

   _____

   _____

3. An example of a virtue is _____.
4. Utilitarianism maintains that what is best for _____ is the best solution.

REFERENCES

BrainyQuote. (2012a). *Confucius quotes*. Retrieved from http://www.brainyquote.com/quotes/authors/c/confucius.html#ixzzloqsbChul

BrainyQuote. (2012b). *Socrates quotes*. Retrieved from http://www.brainyquote.com/quotes/authors/s/socrates.html

Fieser, J. (2003). Ethics. *The Internet Encyclopedia of Philosphy*. Retrieved from http://www.iep.utm.edu/ethics

Mack, P. (2004). Utiliatarian ethics in healthcare. *International Journal of the Computer, the Internet and Management, 12*(3), 63–72.

Pima County, Arizona. (n.d). *Death of Socrates*. Retrieved from http://www.pima.gov/publicdefender/socrates.htm

Tooley, M. (n.d.). *Philosophy 1100—Introduction to ethics*. University of Colorado Boulder. Retrieved from http://spot.colorado.edu/~tooley/Lecture5-EthicalTheories.pdf

Chapter 2

Top Priority: The Patient

We ourselves feel that what we are doing is just a drop in the ocean. But the ocean would be less because of that missing drop.

—Mother Teresa

KEY TERMS

Consent	Informed consent
Contract for care	(or express consent)
Countertransference	Noncompliance
Dignity	Patient Care Partnership
Empathy	Patient's Bill of Rights (PBOR)
Good Samaritan law	Respect
Healthcare consumer	Standard of care
Implied consent	Transference

ESTABLISHING ETHICAL STANDARDS

Dr. William Mayo, founder of the Mayo Clinic, knew how to properly put the patient front and center stage, saying, "The best interest of the patient is the only interest to be considered" (Mayo, 1910). He also believed a patient is "not like a wagon, to be taken apart and repaired in pieces, but should be examined thoroughly and treated as a whole" (Kansas Department of Health and Environment, 2010). Seeing the patient as an individual is essential in performing healthcare services to the highest of standards. After all, no patient, no health care.

A foundation of trust should exist in every healthcare provider–patient relationship. If you do not know the answer to a patient's question, for example, do not just throw an answer out there. You could say something like, "I want to be sure I give you the correct information, so let me research that just to be sure and I will let you know soon." Then follow through with your promise of getting back with an answer soon.

In seeking trust from your patient, you need to hold yourself to the highest of ethical standards. Can you think of gaps where a healthcare professional might fail in doing so? Two examples of high ethical standards follow. Can you think of more?

1. Never let a company's influence or your personal relationships or greed prevent you from putting the patient's best interest first. For example, if a drug representative comes to the clinic where you work often and has forged a close relationship with you and others in the clinic, it should not make you any more likely to prefer that representative's product over another representative's product. The right treatment for the patient should be based solely on what will bring about the best results for that patient.
2. Resources should not be wasted due to professional shortcomings. In other words, do not overuse supplies or use unnecessary supplies in caring for a patient; doing so will contribute to higher medical bills. On the other hand, do not withhold needed items and put your patient at risk.

SEEING RED: RESPECT, EMPATHY, AND DIGNITY IN HEALTH CARE

Though your personal life and your professional life should be kept separate, certainly your values heavily influence your thoughts, words, and actions. The wise healthcare professional knows the worth of putting the patient first and giving every patient, regardless of that patient's appearance, economics, or beliefs, the best of care. Not only is it professionally wise, it is ethically sound. As a college student, you likely know the definition of respect, empathy, and dignity, but it is good to keep their definitions in the forefront of your mind in order to be the most ethical professional possible.

Remembering how you would want to be treated as a patient and understanding patient needs will enhance how you serve patients. This trait is known as **empathy** and is the mark of a top-notch health-care professional.

Respect is another attribute necessary in quality health care. To respect someone is to show that person attention and regard the person's feelings.

Dignity is a bit different from empathy and respect in that it is a result of one or both of the two. In other words, you can show empathy and respect, but not dignity. **Dignity** is a result of another person showing you regard. Specifically, if you show a patient respect, you can empower that person to feel dignity. Dignity varies depending on the receiver, but it certainly is an issue in certain populations, such as with vulnerable populations like the elderly.

Remember that when a patient goes to a healthcare provider for help, he or she probably will not be at a personal best. When you are ill, let's face it, you are probably not at your most personable. Remember that patients may be irritable or withdrawn, or may otherwise behave differently than normal. You, the healthcare professional, will then be called upon to present your highest standard of professionalism by maintaining a spirit of helpfulness, knowledge, and regard for the other person's condition. Professionalism at this level takes practice and determination.

Case Study: Robert Sidakis

You are a medical assistant in the ABC Medical Clinic, where you have served for the past 15 years. Today, you enter the examination room and find Mr. Robert Sidakis waiting. Mr. Sidakis has been a patient of this clinic for more than 20 years. You greet him: "Good morning, Mr. Sidakis. How are we doing today?"

"How am *I* doing today? I'll tell you how I'm doing! I'm sicker than I've ever been and I've been waiting in that waiting room full of coughs, sneezes, and viruses for over two hours and then in this exam room for another hour. I should be treated better than this, and this may be my last visit!"

Knowing that this is not this patient's usual attitude, how would you approach the situation?

In some cases, the patient is noticeably agitated and certainly not in the mood for small talk. Whether or not this is the patient's usual behavior, you are called on through professionalism to put your feelings aside and attend to his or her needs. Your first response should be one of empathy and concern. In the Robert Sidakis case study, you might say, "Mr. Sidakis, I am so sorry. You are a valued patient and we want to make sure you are well taken care of! Let me go ahead and get your vitals so we can start taking care of you right away, then I will check to see what the holdup was."

It may be difficult for you to not become angry when a patient lashes out at you, but as a professional, you will learn that the patient feels bad and not to take it personally. Your top priority every day in your professional life should be the patient's best interest. You are a vital part of the healthcare team, and your knowledge and actions may make either a positive impression or a poor impression on the patient. Which would you prefer? Of course, you would prefer a positive impression.

THE HEALTHCARE CONSUMER

For Your Consideration

The familiar saying goes, "Doctors make the worst patients." Can you think why this could be true and how it can be applied to all healthcare professionals, not just doctors? How can your answer to this question be turned into a positive? How could being a healthcare professional make you a better patient? List your thoughts before reading this section.

As a healthcare professional, you will experience two specific roles: that of the provider and, at some point, that of the healthcare consumer. Anyone seeking professional care or treatment for health is considered a **healthcare consumer**. It is good to be an informed patient; everyone should be. When you do find yourself in the patient role, be sure to ask questions and stay informed; however, do not hinder your healthcare providers from serving you. Remember how it feels to be a patient so that when you are serving patients in a professional role, you will be more likely to deliver the highest standard of care. After all, healthcare facilities deal with two sensitive issues: a patient's health and his or her money.

Health care is one of the most expensive purchases you can make. Consider this: The average daily cost of a hospital stay in the United States is a minimum (on average) of $5,000. In the western United States, that cost averages more than $7,000, the cost of staying in a very luxurious hotel with various amenities. Now, compare that to a day at Disney World with an overnight stay on the property plus meals, which totals $700 (and that includes the price of an airline ticket). Patients with health insurance might have to pay only 20% of that $7,000, which comes out to $1,400, still twice the amount of a day and accommodations at Disney World. Why all this talk about pricing? It is to drive home the point that patient care is expensive, so the healthcare consumer expects, rightfully so, to get the highest standard of care.

Table 2-1 shows the average lengths of stay by U.S. region, the average charges to the patient, and the costs of care (Becker's Hospital

Table 2-1 Hospital Average Length of Stay, Charges, and Costs by Region

U.S. Region	Length of Stay (days)	Average Charges	Average Costs
Northeast	5.1	$27,734	$9,917
Midwest	4.3	$21,522	$8,292
South	4.6	$23,695	$7,888
West	4.3	$35,721	$9,604
Overall	**4.6**	**$26,120**	**$8,692**

Courtesy of: Becker's Hospital Review.

Review, 2009). Remember, a charge may dramatically differ from what is actually collected from the patient and/or insurance company.

ETHICAL CONSIDERATIONS IN HEALTHCARE PROVIDER–PATIENT RELATIONSHIPS

The relationship you have with patients is a fragile one. You want to provide the highest standard of care, but what does that mean? In the healthcare industry, **standard of care** refers to the attention given to a task (with a patient) that would reasonably be expected to be given by anyone in a similar situation. This term is more a legal term than a medical one, and how it is judged is the foundation of many legal actions against medical professionals.

When a person goes to a hospital, clinic, or any type of healthcare service facility, that person is seeking out help for some type of problem or concern. In seeking help, the patient should come to trust the healthcare team. In a professional relationship, special attention is given to the patient as an individual, and lines are clearly drawn about what is and what is not appropriate behavior in this healthcare provider–patient relationship. The following are some guidelines of which you should be aware in maintaining a professional relationship with your patients:

1. Remember, care is built on trust, and when you fail to deliver high-quality care, you violate that trust.
2. Leave the room when a patient is undressing for an examination unless the patient needs assistance. If this is the case, have at least one other healthcare professional present to assist the patient.
3. Do not use inappropriate language, such as telling jokes with sexual content, and never use racial slurs.
4. When a physician is conducting an intimate examination (such as a Pap smear), there should be at least one other healthcare professional present. Conversations should be limited to informing the patient of what is being done during these types of examinations or treatments.

5. Listen to the patient without judging. If it is a problem to the patient, then it is a problem, regardless of your personal opinions. Listening closely may give you information that will help in the diagnosis and successful treatment of the patient.

6. Be careful not to overstep personal boundaries. You want your patient to feel respected and cared for, but you should do so on a professional level. Questions about marital status, sexual orientation, religion, and other highly sensitive areas should be avoided unless they directly relate to the medical concern. Be sure to make it clear that you are there to give the best health care possible on a professional basis.

7. Sexual contact (even flirting) is unprofessional and unethical, and should be completely avoided. Even outside of the healthcare setting you are a healthcare provider, so any such conduct with patients is forbidden. (This subject is further discussed in the Transference section that follows.)

8. It is highly unethical to visit with a patient outside of the health-care setting, including the patient coming to your home or you going to the patient's home. Of course, there is the rare occasion when the physician makes a house call, but this is a professional call and is not the same as a personal visit.

9. Never make promises to a patient. This is not only unethical but illegal. For example, a patient has just been diagnosed with cancer. You say to the patient, "Don't worry, we are going to fix this." Whether or not you realize it, you have just made a promise, and if you do not keep that promise, you can be sued for not delivering on your promise.

TRANSFERENCE

The healthcare provider–patient relationship comes in different forms, which are as unique as the people involved. A patient may even retain feelings or attitudes associated with childhood, which may surface during treatment and may be transferred onto the healthcare provider. This phenomenon is known as **transference**.

Case Study: Susan Walters and Dr. Henson

Susan Walters has been extremely fatigued lately and cannot understand why. She has not changed anything in her usual diet, exercise, or stress level. She schedules an appointment with family physician Dr. George Henson. Dr. Henson notices during the physical examination that Susan is overly tense; also, she is irritable during the consultation portion of the office visit. Dr. Henson, a kind and patient physician, takes the time to talk with the patient and learns that as a child, she was raped by two uncles. Thus, Dr. Henson realizes that Susan's behavior toward him is due to transference of her childhood tragedy. Dr. Henson uses this information to come to some stunning conclusions about Susan's health, namely that she has been suppressing her reaction from the rape incidents and they have taken a toll on her health some 25 years later. Transference, though unfortunate, can help the healthcare provider in addressing patient needs.

How often do you think transference occurs with patients? What are some strategies healthcare professionals should use in working with these cases?

Though transference is usually associated with the patient developing feelings of love or sexual attraction to the professional, it can involve other feelings, such as those exhibited in Susan's case study.

Transference does not always originate with the patient. When the provider experiences feelings for the patient that are out of the norm, such as love, anger, or any other emotion, this is known as **countertransference**. It is obvious that a healthcare provider should never engage in a personal relationship with a patient. The primary responsibility for honoring healthcare provider–patient boundaries is in the hands of the healthcare provider. What can you do to be sure these boundaries are never crossed?

CONTRACTS AND CONSENT

The healthcare provider–patient relationship is a type of contract. For purposes of this discussion, we will define a **contract for care** as an agreement that creates a relationship where the healthcare provider is to provide care to the patient.

Consent is a patient's agreement to treatment. Unlike the contract, consent is for specific health care, such as a consultation or an injection. Consent comes in two forms: (1) informed and (2) implied.

Informed consent occurs when the physician explains the treatment or procedure(s) and the patient or patient representative agrees to have them performed. The consent can be verbal, but it is usually written. This type of consent is most protective of the physician's liability. Another term for informed consent is express consent. An example of informed consent would be when a physician tells a patient she has thyroid cancer and consults with her about treatment options, possible side effects, and other important information. The informed consent could be in the form of a written statement signed by the patient (and sometimes the physician as well) declaring understanding.

Implied consent occurs when a patient's behavior suggests compliance. For example, a nurse comes into the examination room and says, "The doctor has ordered a shot of antibiotic for your sinus infection." If the patients rolls up his or her sleeve to accept the shot, then the patient has given implied consent. This type of consent is more passive, while informed is more active. In emergency situations, such as a car wreck, consent by accident victims is considered implied.

In these emergency situations, the **Good Samaritan law** protects the healthcare provider from being sued when performing medical care in good faith (New York State Department of Health, 2009). The Good Samaritan law protects healthcare providers and even, in some cases, other providers, such as those who provide free medical services at clinics. The law got its name from a story in the Bible (Luke 10:25–37), where a passerby helped a robbery victim even though he did not know the victim. It turned out that the two men were actually enemies because of their differing religious beliefs. However, while others passed by and did not help the victim, the Good Samaritan tended to his needs without bias or fear of repercussions.

According to Robert L. Payton, "Every state in the U.S. now has some version of a 'Good Samaritan Law' providing immunity from liability to those who try to help (some state laws only protect doctors)." Payton also reports that some of these laws include a "duty to assist" statute, making it a crime (misdemeanor) for a healthcare professional to see an accident and not stop to offer assistance (Payton, n.d.).

CAN A PHYSICIAN "FIRE" A PATIENT?

The wise healthcare consumer knows that he or she may seek other treatment if the physician is not meeting standards or producing results. However, a physician, in certain situations, also has the legal and moral right to "fire" (release) a patient.

In June 1996, the American Medical Association (AMA) issued *Opinion 8.115—Termination of the Physician–Patient Relationship:*

> Physicians have an obligation to support continuity of care for their patients. While physicians have the option of withdrawing from a case, they cannot do so without giving notice to the patient, the relatives, or responsible friends sufficiently long in advance of withdrawal to permit another medical attendant to be secured. (AMA, 1996)

Contracts that are violated may be terminated. Patients may be dismissed from a certain physician's care due to:

- **Noncompliance:** Noncompliance is when a patient does not follow a doctor's advice. For example, if a patient seeks care for diabetes but clearly is not following the treatment plan set forth and continues to decline in health, the physician has the legal right to release the patient from care.
- **Insurance plan participation:** Physicians often must decide which insurance plans to accept and which ones not to accept. In such cases, the physician may with due cause dismiss a patient. Other times, a physician may be restricted from

participating in an insurance plan (such as Medicare) due to not following plan directions properly or due to fraud.

- **Patient's failure to keep appointments**: When a patient consistently shows up late for an appointment or does not show up at all, he or she may be released from care.
- **Nonpayment:** If a patient does not pay for service, he or she may be released.

Trivia Quest

The American Hospital Association developed the **Patient's Bill of Rights (PBOR)** in 1973, with a revision in 1992. In 2003, the PBOR was replaced with the Patient Care Partnership.

THE PATIENT CARE PARTNERSHIP

The American Hospital Association developed the **Patient Care Partnership** as a guide for patients to better understand their rights and responsibilities when receiving medical care during a hospital stay. The document also addresses financial aspects of patient care, confidentiality, and the fact that patients have choices in their own medical care.

PUTTING IT ALL TOGETHER

As stated at the beginning of this chapter, no patient, no health care. Though the healthcare professional may bring a personal approach to caring for a patient, it is always the patient's best interest that should prevail. There will likely be plenty of times when you will provide care for a patient who is different from you in appearance and/or beliefs, but that should not prevent you from giving that patient the very best of healthcare services.

The patient has certain rights, including respect, empathy, and dignity (RED). Other rights can be reviewed in the U.S. Government Bill of Rights under the Affordable Care Act. Here, you will find information that will empower the consumer to receive the highest standard of care—something for which you should always strive. Included under ethical and legal considerations are the issues of consent and contract. To fully understand one's obligation to the patient, the healthcare provider should have a working understanding of the Good Samaritan law and reasons a physician can release a patient from care.

The main idea in this chapter is that the best care of the patient is, and should *always* be, the first concern of the healthcare professional. If you find yourself not placing the patient first, you need to immediately check yourself and change your actions to do so.

CHAPTER CHECKUP

Fill-in-the-Blank

1. An agreement that creates a relationship where the healthcare provider is to provide care to the patient is a _____ _____ _____ .

2. When a patient grants an expression of agreement to treatment, it is called _____ .

3. Another word for informed consent is _____ consent.

4. No patient, no _____ .

In Your Own Words

1. Discuss the similarities and differences between respect, empathy, and dignity.

2. How should you treat a patient who is being rude and/or impatient?

Multiple Choice

1. The Patient's Bill of Rights was developed by U.S. government officials in 2010 as part of the:

   A. American Medical Association.
   B. Patient's Rights Constitution.
   C. Affordable Care Act.

2. The phenomenon in which a patient retains feelings or attitudes associated with childhood that may surface during treatment and may be transferred to the healthcare provider is:

   A. transference.
   B. transmitted emotion.
   C. transmission.

REFERENCES

American Medical Association. (1996, June). *AMA code of medical ethics.* Retrieved from http://www.ama-assn.org/ama/pub/physician-resources/medical-ethics/code-medical-ethics/opinion8115.page

Becker's Hospital Review. (2009, July 28). *Hospital average length of stay, charges and costs by region.* Retrieved from http://www.beckershospitalreview.com/lists-and-statistics/hospital-average-length-of-stay-charges-and-costs-by-region.html

Kansas Department of Health and Environment. (2010). *Annual risk management report for 2010.* Retrieved from http://www.kdheks.gov/bhfr/download/2010_RM_Annual_Rpt.pdf

Mayo, W. (1910). *The best interest of the patient.* Mayo Clinic. Retrieved from http://www.mayoclinic.org/tradition-heritage-artifacts/44-2.html

New York State Department of Health. (2009, February 3). *Public health law article 30.* Retrieved from http://www.health.ny.gov/nysdoh/ems/art30.htm

Payton, R. L. (n.d.). *Faith groups.* Learning to Give. Retrieved from http://learningtogive.org/faithgroups/phil_in_america/philanthropy_good.asp

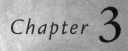

Chapter 3

Vulnerable Populations

Until the great mass of the people shall be filled with the sense of responsibility for each other's welfare, social justice can never be attained.

—Helen Keller

IN THIS CHAPTER, YOU WILL LEARN ABOUT:

- Legal and ethical issues surrounding minors
- Legal and ethical issues surrounding elderly populations
- Legal and ethical issues surrounding HIV/AIDS
- Legal and ethical issues surrounding cultural and other differences
- Mandatory reporting

KEY TERMS

Acquired immune deficiency syndrome (AIDS)
Advance directive
Americans With Disabilities Act
Autonomy
Child abuse
Competent
Do not resuscitate (DNR)
Domestic abuse
Elder abuse
Guardian ad litem
Health Insurance Portability and Accountability Act (HIPAA)
HELP model
Human immunodeficiency virus (HIV)
Living will
Mandatory reporting laws
Mature minor doctrine
Medicaid
Medicare
Power of attorney (POA)
Ryan White HIV/AIDS Program
Title X
Withdrawing or withholding treatment

INTRODUCTION

As discussed in the previous chapters, all patients have certain legal and ethical rights. These rights protect the patients from harm and provide them with an ability to make choices. Certain populations, however, are more vulnerable to harm and require greater protection. There are laws directly related to these populations that guide healthcare professionals in decision-making processes. In addition, there are ethical situations that apply specifically to each population. What groups can you think of that might be considered a vulnerable population? In this chapter, you will learn the specifics on vulnerable populations and special considerations for serving them.

MINORS

Legally, in the United States minors are considered anyone younger than 18 years of age. In general, all medical procedures for minors require parental or guardian consent (**Figure 3-1**). However, as healthcare policy moves toward increased patient autonomy, including the rights of patients to be involved in decision-making processes, the rights of minors come into question. Who makes decisions for minors? At what age should minors be allowed to provide or refuse consent? What happens if the minor does not agree with the decision of a parent or guardian? Or, if a minor wishes to seek medical advice without a parent,

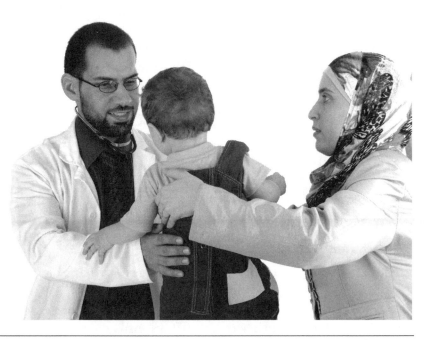

Figure 3-1 A child receiving care from a physician.

should this be allowed? There are not always clear-cut answers to these questions, but certain laws and ethical principles can help healthcare professionals decide on an appropriate course of action.

Historically, the age of **autonomy** has been 18. Autonomy is a person's ability to make decisions concerning his or her own personal business, including health care. Because minors are not considered legally old enough to provide informed consent, a parent or guardian steps in to provide consent. This means that anyone younger than 18 years of age needs someone older to act as a surrogate decision maker to assume responsibility for doing what is best for the minor. If the minor does not have a parent, such as in the case of a child whose parents have died or a child in the custody of the state (as with foster care), the courts will appoint a **guardian ad litem**. This person acts as the legal guardian for all decision-making processes, including decisions regarding health care. There are also cases where parents assume the role of guardian ad litem for disabled children after they reach the age of majority or for their elderly parents who are no longer considered **competent**.

Reasonable and rational parents (or guardians) base their healthcare decisions on family values, resources, and needs. Not all families will make the same decisions, because they have different values, different financial resources, and different needs. As healthcare professionals, our duty is to explain the various choices available and respect decisions made—regardless of personal opinions. We might not always agree with a family's decisions, but our role is to advise, not judge.

A healthcare professional will sometimes feel that family decisions conflict with the best interests of the child. These instances may result from religious and cultural differences, and may involve minors who are facing an untimely death. Certain religions and cultures have strict guidelines regarding medical issues. For example, families that practice Jehovah's Witness see blood transfusions as a violation of their religious practice. The Jehovah's Witness believes that any blood that leaves one body should not be placed in another body and, further, that any blood that leaves the body should be discarded. Jehovah's Witnesses will accept other types of fluid infusion, such as medications, just not blood. To follow this type of religious policy is an acceptable decision for an informed adult, but withholding a lifesaving procedure from a minor because of parental religious convictions is generally found to be an ethical and legal dilemma.

Case in Point: Blood Transfusions and Jehovah's Witnesses

At 2 years of age, Johnny was diagnosed with acute lymphoblastic leukemia. Johnny's parents were practicing Jehovah's Witnesses who refused all blood transfusions (McNeil, 1997). Johnny's parents were willing to try other therapies, but not any that required blood products. Jehovah's Witnesses, as a religious group, refuse blood products based on strict observance of certain laws in the Bible. The physicians chose to work with Johnny's parents and offered other remedies to replace hemoglobin counts that are often lowered during chemotherapy required to treat leukemia. The hospital also chose to obtain a court order allowing them to give Johnny a blood transfusion if his life were threatened. The court based the decision on the 1944 Supreme Court case of Prince vs. Commonwealth of Massachusetts. In that case, the courts ruled that "[t]he right to practice religion freely does not include the liberty to expose . . . a child . . . to ill health or death. Parents may be free to become martyrs themselves. But it does not follow that they are free . . . to make martyrs of their children before the children reach the age of full and legal discretion when they can make the choice for themselves" (*Prince v. Commonwealth of Massachusetts*, 1944).

Unfortunately, at one of Johnny's checkups, it was decided that his hemoglobin and platelet counts were dangerously low. Johnny was given a blood and platelet transfusion against the wishes of his parents. Only one transfusion was needed and Johnny remains in remission from leukemia. His parents were devastated, but because it was a court decision and not their own, they felt as if they still upheld their religious beliefs.

As the case of Johnny illustrates, healthcare professionals occasionally need to consult the legal system when there are conflicts between the decisions of the parents and what the medical community considers to be in the best interest of the child. In other situations, the outcomes of certain decisions are unknown and thus controversial. For instance, due to religious or personal reasons, some parents might refuse to allow their child to become vaccinated. While healthcare professionals promote the use of vaccines as a benefit to patients and society as a whole, legally the parents have a right to refuse this medical procedure for their children. Most states require children to be fully vaccinated before they can enter the public school system, but parents with religious or secular convictions can opt out of this requirement. The controversy around this issue continues as some parents who opted out due to concerns that vaccinations might be linked to development disorders, such as autism, learn that the research was fraudulent. One difference between allowing parents to opt out of vaccinations and refusing lifesaving medical procedures is that once minors reach the age of majority, they can choose to obtain the vaccinations themselves. So far, the overall number of parents opting out of vaccinations is relatively small and has not led to widespread outbreaks of dreaded diseases. However, this is something that healthcare professionals might want to consider as an important area of parental education.

Making choices for infants is another difficult area for healthcare professionals. If a woman goes into labor early, how does the medical community decide which procedures are helpful and which are harmful? A premature infant born at less than 23 weeks' gestation is generally not resuscitated because the medical community agrees that quality of life for the infant would be poor. After 25 weeks, aggressive measures are taken to resuscitate the newborn. Between 23 and 25 weeks, the decision is left up to the parents and medical community based on various factors, including overall health of the newborn, trauma of the birth process, and resources of the family. Asking parents to provide informed consent at this stage is problematic because of traumatic outcomes that are difficult to predict. The parents are asked to either give up a future child or face the possibility of raising a child with developmental and medical difficulties (Ravitsky, Fiester, & Caplan, 2009).

Case in Point: Gregory Messenger

In Michigan, a man was accused of manslaughter after removing his son from a respirator that was preserving the premature infant's life. Gregory Messenger and his wife were concerned that the baby, who was born 15 weeks premature, would have severe brain damage. The infant had been given a 50% chance of survival at the time of birth. Messenger and his wife had told doctors not to place the infant on life support, but the doctor in charge ordered a respirator to be used if the infant was active after delivery. Messenger was acquitted (Man acquitted in death of infant, 1995).

In other cases, the parent or guardian might have a difficult time making decisions regarding options for their minor, especially when a minor requires life support. Making the decision to withdraw or withhold life support is never easy for a parent. Healthcare professionals may be asked to provide guidance when it comes to this type of decision. It is always important to consider several factors, including the reason for the life support (e.g., tragic accident vs. chronic illness).

So far we have discussed the decision-making process for young minors who depend solely on their parents or guardians for healthcare-related decisions. In some cases, however, older minors may not agree with the decisions of their parents or guardians. At what age do minors have the capacity to make their own decisions? The answer varies from state to state and depends on certain variables, such as chosen procedures and medical conditions.

Typically, most states consider anyone 12 years of age and younger incapable of making informed medical decisions. Once the minor becomes a teenager, the courts consider various factors. For example, many states allow minors to obtain contraceptives and prenatal care without parental consent or notification. **Title X**, a federal family planning program, specifically provides these services to minors. Several attempts have been made to make parental notification or consent a requirement for obtaining the services, but so far these attempts have failed. In most states, however, laws require parental consent and/or notification of at least one parent before a minor can have an abortion. The U.S. Supreme Court does grant minors a limited amount of privacy when it comes to abortion procedures. The recognition of this privacy allows for courts to bypass parental consent if it is decided that the minor is mature enough and understands the risks involved.

Other circumstances allow for a waiver of parental consent for minors. These include emergency situations in which it is assumed the parents would provide consent, sexual abuse instances where the parent is suspected to be involved in the abuse, and mental health or substance abuse services (minors can seek treatment without notifying parents). Finally, most states allow anyone older than 12 years of age to be tested and treated for sexually transmitted diseases, including HIV, without parental notification or consent. Some states do require notification, and some states restrict the treatment allowed without parental consent. As a healthcare professional, it is important to know the laws specific to the state in which you are licensed.

While family planning decisions are a common ethical and legal issue for minors, there are other situations in which minors and parents/guardians might not agree on the treatment options. For instance, minors with a chronic illness are often better suited to make medical decisions because of their experience. However, it is also important to consider the other factors, including stage of development, cognitive and emotional ability, and environment.

When a healthcare professional is working with minors, all of these factors must be considered in determining how much the minor should be told about treatment options and how much autonomy he or she will be granted in the decision-making process. In some states, the **mature minor doctrine** provides greater autonomy to minors older than 16 years of age who understand and consent to relatively simple medical procedures. This doctrine is a legal concept used by the courts, but a few states have passed it as a statute. Even if healthcare professionals consider these factors and believe a minor to be able to provide informed consent, the parents might not agree. If parents and minors do not agree on the course of medical action to be taken, the legal system may be called upon to intervene.

Case in Point: Starchild Abraham Cherrix

Sixteen-year-old Starchild Abraham Cherrix was diagnosed with Hodgkin disease. After an initial regimen of chemotherapy, he refused any further treatments, stating that he wished to try alternative medicine instead. His parents supported this decision, which led to an accusation of neglect. A juvenile court found Cherrix's parents guilty of medical neglect and required that he return to conventional treatment. An appeal to a circuit court resulted in a reverse of this decision and allowed Cherrix and his family to work with an oncologist (a doctor specializing in cancer treatments) interested in alternative cancer treatments (Hester, n.d.). After this case was settled, the state of Virginia added Abraham's Law to permit parents to "refuse medical treatment or to choose alternative treatments for children aged 14 to 17 with a life-threatening medical condition, if the teenager seems to be mature, both the parents and the child have considered the treatment options available to them, and all agree that their choice is in the child's best interest" (63.2-100 of the Code of Virginia).

ELDERLY PATIENTS

Advance directives are legal documents outlining the health and welfare wishes of a patient if that patient is unable to communicate for himself or herself or is no longer considered competent. A **do not resuscitate (DNR)** order informs healthcare professionals that patients do not want extreme measures taken to save their life during cardiac arrest. A **living will** is a legal document that indicates whether a patient wants to be placed on life-prolonging machines (also known as life support) if they are unable to communicate for themselves.

A **power of attorney (POA)** is a written document that legally allows someone to make decisions on another's behalf. There are several different types of POAs, including, but not limited to, healthcare proxy, healthcare agent, healthcare surrogate, and POA for health care. The terms and definitions vary from state to state, and it is usually best to obtain information on advance directives from your local hospital, as they will have documents that comply with state laws and regulations.

Advance directives must be created by a competent adult prior to the illness or injury. If an elderly patient has an advance directive in his or her medical record, this form will direct the healthcare professionals in decisions regarding medical care. It is important to note that in emergency situations, healthcare professionals might make decisions without the benefit of an existing advance directive or family input.

If the patient does not have an advance directive, then the medical professionals and family members are left with the responsibility of determining what is best for the patient in cases of emergencies or serious illness. In these cases, the medical professional will most likely use the ethical principle of beneficence (do no harm) in making medical decisions. This can be a challenge as the medical team decides whether certain types of treatment generally provided to cure younger patients might actually cause more harm for elderly patients. For example, if a 45-year-old man requires bypass surgery to survive, the medical team will not likely question performing this procedure. However, if an 85-year-old man requires the same surgery, the medical team might deem it more harmful than beneficial.

One of the biggest ethical and legal issues surrounding the elderly is the issue of competence. Competence generally refers to an individual's ability to make decisions necessary to live independently. An individual can be declared incompetent, which indicates an inability to make those necessary decisions, at any age. If a person suffers a severe head trauma, for example, and is left with major brain damage, he or she might be considered incompetent (**Figure 3-2**). In the case of the elderly, incompetence might be associated with certain diseases,

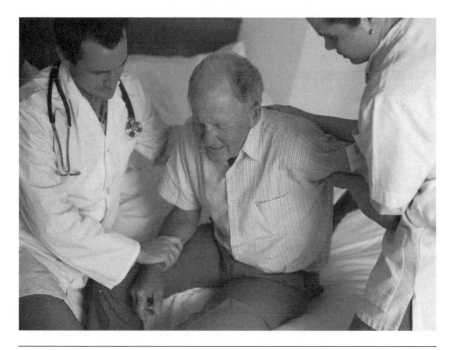

Figure 3-2 An elderly patient with a medical assistant.

such as Alzheimer's disease or dementia, but sometimes an elderly person might lose critical thinking skills simply due to aging or over-all diminished health. At this point, a family member or a healthcare professional working closely with the patient might need to appoint a guardian to make medical decisions for that patient.

Making medical decisions for an elderly parent or close friend is not always a simple task (**Figure 3-3**). The decision to **withdraw or withhold medical treatment** is often very emotional. Medical pro-fessionals must always take time to explain the options and provide as much information as possible during the decision-making pro-cess. For example, a grieving daughter might need to be reminded that cancer is the ultimate cause of death of a loved one, not the removal of the breathing tube. In other instances, the healthcare professional needs to respect the choices of family members even if they disagree.

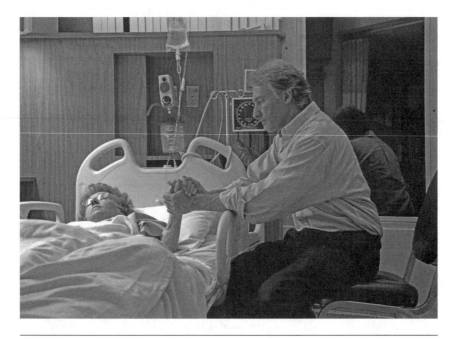

Figure 3-3 Making medical decisions for an elderly parent or close friend is difficult.

Your job as a healthcare professional is to serve the patient and his or her best interests, not to make healthcare or any other decisions for the patient. For example, an elderly patient might refuse chemotherapy or a difficult surgery because the patient feels he or she has lived a good life and would prefer to die without medical intervention. At all times, a healthcare professional must make sure a competent patient's wishes are respected.

Elderly patients are often faced with increased healthcare expenses. While some patients have adequate insurance coverage and financial resources, others will depend on Medicare. **Medicare** is a federally sponsored program that provides healthcare coverage for adults 65 years of age and older, as well as some adults younger than 65 years of age with certain disabilities.

Medicare coverage is divided into several parts. Part A helps cover the cost of inpatient care in hospitals, skilled nursing facilities, hospice, and home health care. The coverage of Part A generally comes at no cost to the patient because the patient and/or the patient's spouse has already contributed income tax dollars toward the Medicare program. Those who do not qualify for Part A for free can choose from various plans that have a monthly premium associated with them. Part B covers other doctor expenses, including some preventive care, medical equipment, and rehabilitation services. There is usually a monthly premium associated with Part B. Those who are required to pay a monthly premium for Part A also pay a monthly premium for Part B. Parts C and D are optional and provide additional coverage, including prescription drugs. Because the Medicare program is federally funded, the benefits are provided equally across the nation.

Some low-income elderly patients may qualify for Medicaid. **Medicaid** provides assistance to low-income individuals and families to pay for health care. The funding for Medicaid comes from the federal government, but the states choose who qualifies and how to distribute the coverage (Centers for Medicaid and Medicare, 2011).

It is important to note that a physician is not required to accept Medicaid or Medicare. If the physician does not accept these government-funded programs, then the patient must either pay out of pocket for the service or seek another healthcare provider. Since the cost of health care is generally beyond what many patients can afford, the refusal to accept Medicare or Medicaid patients is met with some controversy. There are those who question the ethics of this policy—especially in small communities where the choice of healthcare providers is limited. On the other hand, the federal government is allowed to set limits on how much healthcare providers can receive for services provided, and some healthcare providers feel that the rate of reimbursement is not sufficient and thus choose not to accept patients who use Medicare or Medicaid. Additionally, if a facility has been penalized for Medicare or Medicaid fraud, the facility may no longer be allowed to provide services to Medicare and/or Medicaid patients.

HIV/AIDS PATIENTS

Certain communicable diseases cause more public health issues than others. For example, the polio outbreak resulted in mandatory vaccinations as a necessary means to prevent future outbreaks. In the same manner, the HIV/AIDS epidemic of the 1980s resulted in certain laws and ethical principles necessary to protect patients with the disease. Because HIV/AIDS comes with a unique stigma, public health officials realized that these laws were necessary to ensure that efforts at testing, prevention and treatment were not hampered in any way. In addition, the laws attempt to prevent discrimination against people living with HIV/AIDS.

HIV is an abbreviation for the **human immunodeficiency virus**. This virus attacks cells in the body that are responsible for fighting infection and disease, leaving the patient vulnerable to future diseases and making HIV impossible to fight. Over time, HIV infection may lead to AIDS, which stands for **acquired immune deficiency syndrome**. AIDS is the final stage for HIV patients. At this point, the body is unable to naturally fight infections, which leaves patients prone to developing illnesses that people with weakened immune systems are unable to fight, such as pneumonia and certain cancers. HIV is spread through some bodily fluids, including blood, semen, breast milk, vaginal fluids, and rectal mucus. Other bodily fluids, such as urine and fecal matter, can contain the HIV virus, but unless it is mixed with additional bodily fluids, such as blood, it is not generally enough to spread the virus. It is possible for a person who comes in contact with an HIV-infected bodily fluid to get the virus if that bodily fluid is transmitted into his or her body. HIV is generally transmitted during the following activities:

- Sexual contact
- Pregnancy
- Childbirth
- Breastfeeding
- Injected drug use
- Occupational exposure
- Blood transfusion
- Organ transplant

Healthcare professionals are at a greater risk for occupational exposure to HIV because they often are exposed to bodily fluids. Healthcare professionals have contracted the HIV virus through needlesticks and splashes of bodily fluids into their eyes, mouth, or open sores. Therefore, it is important for healthcare professionals to take extra precautions, such as gloves and masks, to avoid exposure to HIV (and other communicable diseases).

The fear of contracting HIV from a patient or coworkers has created a stigma around the diseases that can lead to discrimination. Certain laws protect people living with HIV, including the **Americans With Disabilities Act (ADA)**. Discrimination based on disabilities is unlawful under the ADA. The Supreme Court ruled that HIV infection meets the definition of disability and is therefore covered, which also extends to other state and federal laws. The **Health Insurance Portability and Accountability Act (HIPAA)** has also helped in the prevention of discrimination against HIV/AIDS patients by keeping their medical condition confidential. If individuals living with HIV/AIDS feel that their privacy rights have been violated, they may be eligible to file a complaint through the Office of Civil Rights. HIPAA regulations provide certain protections for people with HIV/AIDS:

- They limit the ability of insurance companies to exclude patients from coverage if they have a preexisting condition (e.g., HIV).
- They prevent group health plans from denying coverage or charging additional fees based on preexisting conditions, including those of family members.
- They guarantee certain small business employers the right to purchase health insurance.
- They guarantee that employers and individuals who purchase health insurance can renew the coverage, regardless of health conditions.

In addition to protection against discrimination, there is federal legislation that attempts to meet the unmet health needs of people living with HIV/AIDS. The **Ryan White HIV/AIDS Program** is a federal program administered by the Health Resources and Services

Administration. It focuses on providing funding for health care and support services to patients with HIV/AIDS.

Case in Point: Ryan White

In 1984, at 13 years of age, Ryan White was diagnosed with AIDS. Other than being a hemophiliac, most would say he had led a normal life. When the diagnosis was pronounced, Ryan found himself in the sweeping storm of a political controversy and media attention. At that time, AIDS was still new to most people and there was little to no education about the condition.

Ryan White and his mother fought AIDS-related discrimination and helped start promotion of AIDS awareness and education. They tirelessly fought for Ryan's rights as an AIDS patient to attend school and have accessibility to health care. Incredibly, this child led the way to educating people around the world about AIDS and equality of health care.

Ryan's story has touched many, and in his honor the Ryan White CARE (Comprehensive AIDS Resources Emergency) Act was first signed into law in May 1996 by then-President Bill Clinton. Since then, it has been reauthorized four times (1996, 2000, 2006, and 2009), exhibiting the commitment to the legacy of Ryan White. It is now called the Ryan White HIV/AIDS Program.

Sadly, Ryan never got to see the act signed into legislation. He died 6 months before the initial legislation was signed (Health Resources and Services Administration, n.d.).

AIDS is a disease—not a dirty word.
—Ryan White

Federal laws are written to protect patients with HIV/AIDS from discrimination and to ensure that they receive appropriate treatment. Certain laws also require efforts toward preventing the spread of the disease itself. Once a patient is diagnosed with HIV, he or she has a legal and ethical responsibility to inform others. Most states allow doctors to inform the infected patient's spouse. Generally, the doctor will allow the patient time to inform the spouse, but the doctor has a legal responsibility to do so if the patient is unwilling. Doctors legally cannot contact other non-spousal sexual partners, so most states require that all HIV-positive patients inform past, present, and future sexual partners, as well as current healthcare providers. The local health department can notify sexual or needle-sharing partners that they may have been exposed to HIV without releasing the name of the contact. Once a person tests positive for HIV, this information is shared with the public health department, but names and other identifying information are kept confidential. Besides past sexual or needle-sharing partners and current healthcare providers, HIV-positive patients are not required to share their status with anyone else—including their employer or coworkers.

Currently, the Centers for Disease Control and Prevention requires healthcare professionals to disclose their HIV status to patients. This policy is considered controversial by some because there have been only a limited number of instances when healthcare professionals have infected patients. However, as long as the risk for exposure exists, healthcare professionals have a legal and ethical obligation to disclose their HIV status to patients (AIDS.gov).

Case in Point: Doe vs. Medlantic Health Care Group (2003)

John Doe (plaintiff) chose not to tell his employer, a cleaning company that provided services to the U.S. Department of State, that he was HIV-positive. A coworker at the State Department, Tijuana Goldring, also worked part-time as a receptionist at the Washington Health Center, which was owned by the Medlantic Health Care Group (defendant). During a checkup at the Washington Health Center, Doe stopped by to say hello to Goldring. Goldring asked for the spelling of Doe's last name so

visitation rights of same-sex partners. In 2010, President Obama issued a memorandum addressing this issue (Obama, 2012). He recommended that all healthcare facilities allow patients to designate and not deny visitation privileges on the basis of race, color, national origin, religion, sex, sexual orientation, gender identity, or disability. Some states have already adopted this policy, and many will most likely follow. Allowing patients to have designated visitors provides comfort during a stressful time. If these visitations are restricted or denied, the patient might lose a necessary advocate.

MANDATORY REPORTING

Vulnerable populations are often at a greater risk of being abused. Healthcare professionals should always be on the lookout for any signs of neglect or abuse when treating all of their patients, but vulnerable populations deserve special attention. There are specific laws regarding abuse of children and elderly persons. The laws requiring healthcare professionals to report suspected cases of abuse are known as **mandatory reporting laws**. These laws vary from state to state, but in general anyone involved in education, health care, or social work must complete training sessions regarding mandatory reporting.

Child abuse is physical, sexual, or emotional mistreatment or the neglect of a child. Any questionable injury of children must be reported, as must signs of neglect. Physicians and other healthcare professionals can be held responsible if they do not report cases of child abuse. On the other hand, if you are acting in the best interest of a child when you report suspected abuse, you cannot be held responsible if you are wrong. In other words, the healthcare professional cannot be sued for making a report regarding child abuse. Most states require that suspected cases of abuse be reported orally followed by a written report. Many states now require reporting of suspected child abuse from anyone, no matter their occupation. In these states, a person who suspects child abuse but does not report it can be held legally responsible for not doing so.

Elder abuse includes intentional harm, neglect, exploitation, and abandonment of persons 60 years of age and older. This type of mandatory reporting is more commonly encountered by healthcare professionals who work in nursing homes or skilled nursing facilities.

Healthcare professionals working in all fields should watch for signs of abuse and neglect when dealing with elderly patients. Elderly patients are also protected from abusive healthcare workers. For example, a recent case involved nursing aides who inappropriately touched elderly patients. They were eventually charged with elder abuse.

Domestic abuse involves willful intimidation, assault, or other abusive behavior committed by one family member or intimate partner against another. These cases are often difficult to confirm, but if a healthcare professional suspects that a patient is involved in a domestic abuse situation, he or she should report these suspicions to the proper authorities **(Figure 3-5)**. Reporting guidelines vary from state to state but generally include notification of a social worker or supervisor.

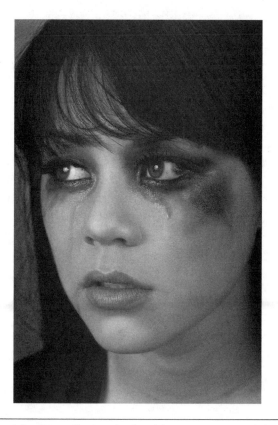

Figure 3-5 Healthcare professionals should report suspected domestic abuse to the proper authorities.

PUTTING IT ALL TOGETHER

As healthcare professionals, it is important to be aware of vulnerable populations, as well as the laws and ethical considerations that surround them. Knowing more about these populations provides an opportunity to meet their needs in the best way possible.

CHAPTER CHECKUP

Fill-in-the-Blank

1. _____ is a person's ability to make decisions concerning his or her own well-being, including health care.
2. In some states, the _____ _____ _____ provides greater autonomy to minors over older than 16 years of age who understand and consent to relatively simple medical procedures.
3. _____ generally refers to an individual's ability to make decisions necessary to live independently.
4. HIV is an abbreviation for the _____ _____ _____.
5. The _____ _____ _____ _____ is a federal program administered by the Health Resources and Services Administration. It focuses on providing funding for health care and support services to patients with HIV/AIDS.
6. The laws requiring healthcare professionals to report suspected cases of abuse are known as _____ _____ _____.

True/False

1. Historically, the age of autonomy has been 21 years.
2. A guardian ad litem is appointed by the courts.
3. Medicare is a federally sponsored program providing healthcare coverage for adults 60 years of age and older.
4. Medicaid provides assistance to low-income individuals and families to pay the cost of health care.
5. Elder abuse includes intentional harm, neglect, exploitation, and abandonment of persons 60 years of age and older.

Discussion

1. What are four ways in which HIV is generally transmitted?
2. When a patient is diagnosed with HIV, whom is he or she required to inform?
3. What vulnerable populations do you think you will interact with as a healthcare professional?
4. What is the HELP model?
5. What types of suspected abuse are mandatory reporters required to report?

REFERENCES

Aids.gov. Retrieved from http://www.aids.gov/

Centers for Medicaid and Medicare. (2011). *What is Medicare?* Retrieved from http://www.medicare.gov/Publications/Pubs/pdf/11306.pdf

Connor, V. (2012). The HELP model.

Doe v. Medlantic Health Care Group, Inc. 814 A.2d 939 (DC Ct. App. 2003).

Hester, D. (n.d.). Abraham Cherrix. *Pediatrics Ethics Consortium.* Retrieved from http://www.pediatricethics.org/index.php?option=com_content&view=article&id=111&I emid=53

Health Resources and Services Administration, (n.d.). *Who was Ryan White?* Retrieved from http://hab.hrsa.gov/abouthab/ryanwhite.html

McNeil, S. (1997). Johnny's story: Transfusing a Jehovah's Witness. *Life and Health Library.* Retrieved from http://findarticles.com/p/articles/mi_m0FSZ/is_n3_v23/ai_n18607405/

Obama, B. (2010). Presidential memorandum—Hospital visitation. Retrieved from http://www.whitehouse.gov/the-press-office/presidential-memorandum-hospital-visitation

Ravitsky, V., Fiester, A., & Caplan, A. (2009). *The Penn Center guide to bioethics* (Kindle edition). New York: Springer Publishing Company.

Prince v. Commonwealth of Massachusetts. 321 US 158 (1944).

Man acquitted in death of infant. (1995). *The New York Times.* Retrieved from http://www.nytimes.com/1995/02/04/us/man-acquitted-in-death-of-infant.html

Chapter 4

Confidentiality

In almost every profession—whether it's law or journalism, finance or medicine or academia or running a small business—people rely on confidential communications to do their jobs. We count on the space of trust that confidentiality provides. When someone breaches that trust, we are all worse off for it.

—Hillary Clinton

IN THIS CHAPTER, YOU WILL LEARN ABOUT:

- The importance of confidentiality in the healthcare industry
- The Health Insurance Portability and Accountability Act (HIPAA)
- Violations of a patient's confidentiality and consequences
- Common breaches of medical information confidentiality
- The Privacy Rule

KEY TERMS

Breach
Confidentiality
Consolidated Omnibus
    Budget Reconciliation Act
    of 1985 (COBRA)
Healthcare Integrity and
    Protection Data Bank
    (HIPDB)
Patient Safety and Quality
    Improvement Act of 2005
    (PSQIA)

Portability
Preexisting condition
Privacy Act of 1974
Privacy Rule
Protected health information
    (PHI)
Release of information

For Your Consideration

Think about secrecy. Honestly, how good are you at keeping secrets? It is tempting to share secrets when "juicy" information is involved, isn't it? As a healthcare professional, you must discipline yourself in keeping confident information in the strictest of secrecy. If this is a challenge for you, remember, practice helps.

CONFIDENTIALITY AS EXPRESSED IN THE HIPPOCRATIC OATH

Even Hippocrates (460–377 BC) realized the value of confidentiality in medicine **(Figure 4-1)**. The following is a portion of the Hippocratic Oath. Please note that there are several versions of the Hippocratic Oath, and this version is often used. What part of this oath addresses confidentiality?

> Whatever houses I may visit, I will come for the benefit of the sick, remaining free of all intentional injustice, of all mischief and in particular of sexual relations with both female and male persons, be they free or slaves.
>
> What I may see or hear in the course of the treatment or even outside of the treatment in regard to the life of men, which on no account one must spread abroad, I will keep to myself, holding such things shameful to be spoken about.

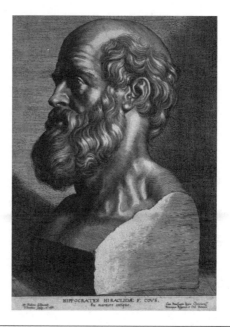

Figure 4-1 Hippocrates.

You were correct if you chose the second paragraph, which states, "I will keep to myself." This passage suggests that no matter the setting, sharing of a person's personal health information is unethical. This statement is just as true and applicable today as the day it was written. Patients have the right to expect that their medical information will be kept confidential, and now, thanks to the Health Insurance Portability and Accountability Act of 1996 (HIPAA), it is illegal to do otherwise.

Protecting a patient's medical information is equivalent to confidentiality. As a healthcare professional, you are entrusted with certain medical information that should be kept in complete confidence. The physician takes the Hippocratic Oath, which includes confidentiality. As part of this duty, the physician must take all necessary steps to secure the patient's medical information. This applies to any healthcare professional.

CONFIDENTIALITY AND THE HEALTHCARE INDUSTRY

For purposes of the healthcare industry, **confidentiality** can be defined as keeping personal medical information private. This includes not only specific conditions and treatments, but the very fact that the person sought treatment in the first place. When a healthcare professional protects a patient's medical information, that professional is showing respect for the patient. When a patient feels respected, he or she could be more likely to trust and more fully cooperate with healthcare providers. This includes giving the physician all information that would help the healthcare team best serve the patient. Confidentiality is not only ethical, it is mandated by law.

Case Study: Dr. George Sheffield

You are a medical assistant in the office of Dr. George Sheffield, a plastic surgeon. Dr. Sheffield is the surgeon to many celebrities, including your sister's favorite actor, Stephen Morris. Mr. Morris has come to Dr. Sheffield's office for consultation about a face-lift. Though you might be excited to serve him and would love to tell your sister, you legally and ethically should not tell your sister that Mr. Morris came to your workplace for a consultation. In fact, telling your sister or anyone that he visited the clinic is illegal since you are clearly violating HIPAA laws and could be penalized (with punishment ranging from fines to imprisonment). Confidentiality is serious business and is to be treated with care and the highest of professionalism. Also remember that although Mr. Morris might be a celebrity, he is not entitled to any better medical care or protection of his medical information than any other patient. In health care, every patient has the right to your best efforts in regard to respect, dignity, and standard of care. Treat each patient as though he or she is the most important of people, celebrity or not.

Beginnings

In the 1960s, the federal government increasingly found it necessary to establish and maintain records of many types. Concerned citizens and legislators wondered about the ways private information could be used by the government. In 1973, the Department of Health, Education, and Welfare (HEW) issued a report titled *Records, Computers, and the Rights of Citizens*. This report caught the attention of legislators, who soon went to work. The **Privacy Act of 1974** (Public Law 93-579) was the result and was signed into law by President Gerald Ford. The Privacy Act is not exclusive to medical information. It addresses a variety of private information, including how social security numbers can be shared. The Privacy Act only applies to U.S. citizens and permanent residents; only these individuals may sue under the statutes of the act. The conversation that preceded and followed the Privacy Act spurred further discussion about privacy, and it would be reasonable to believe that it was, in some ways, the forefather to HIPAA.

Common Breaches of Medical Information Confidentiality

Why in the world is confidentiality so important anyway? First, speaking legally and ethically, a person's healthcare information is private and personal in nature, and every patient has a stake in who views his or her medical record. Secondly, a person might be more likely to seek health care if he or she is assured that medical information will be kept private. By feeling free to be open and honest, the patient reveals accurate information that can help the healthcare team provide the best care.

In everyday professional situations, there are many opportunities for breaches of confidentiality **(Figure 4-2)**. To **breach** means to violate. The following list includes just a few of the ways a healthcare professional fails to guard personal medical information. Can you add others to the list?

1. Perry, a receptionist in a medical office, greets a patient and asks (where others can hear), "Why are you seeing the doctor today?"

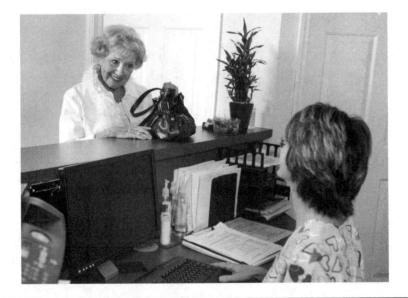

Figure 4-2 Every member of a medical office, from the doctor to the receptionist, is responsible for ensuring patient confidentiality.

2. A sign-in sheet at the front desk of a medical office is in list form, and when a patient comes to sign in, other patients' information (sometimes even including address and phone number) can be openly viewed.
3. A nurse and doctor are in an area near examination rooms. They are discussing the patient they just saw, Maria Fernandez. Patients in the examination rooms, as well as those passing through, can easily hear what is being said concerning Ms. Fernandez.
4. An insurance clerk leaves her computer on while she goes to lunch. In plain sight is the insurance record of Mr. James Foreman. In addition, the screen is visible to those signing in.
5. Mr. Milton McMurray is a night-shift custodian for the medical office of Dr. Jay Smith. Mr. McMurray is the only person in the office at night as he works. Without anyone knowing, he occasionally reads medical records of patients whom he knows. After all, he has to vacuum the carpet in the records storage room and has easy access when he is cleaning.

In Scenario 1, the receptionist may not realize it, but he has just broken patient confidentiality by asking the patient the reason for this office visit. Such information should not be discussed "in earshot" of others. Instead, the receptionist can ask the patient to come around to the side where others cannot hear. Even better, when the patient makes the appointment, the healthcare professional can ask the reason for the visit over the phone so that others do not hear the response. In doing so, the reason for the visit is already stated and does not need to be revisited, especially in a public place such as the reception area of a medical office.

Scenario 2 is a common mistake in medical offices. The best method of patient sign-in is to have stickers on which the patient signs in, and after doing so, the sticker is immediately removed from the sign-in sheet and put on another sheet to document the patient docket of the day. At the end of the day, this list should be filed in a secure location. Many medical office supply companies sell these stickers, so it is easy to access this secure method of patient sign-in.

In Scenario 3, the two healthcare professionals have obviously overlooked the fact that others can hear the confidential patient information they are discussing. This breach can easily be remedied by stepping into the physician's office or other private setting to discuss the case.

Insurance information, such as that presented in Scenario 4, is as confidential as the medical record itself. With that in mind, the insurance clerk must carefully guard insurance information just as the medical staff guards the medical record. To prevent such information from being viewed by others, the insurance clerk should have logged out of her computer before going to lunch. Additionally, the insurance clerk should have an automatic computer save-and-shutoff setting for when the computer is left idol for more than 30 seconds. This can be adjusted within the computer's control panel settings. If you use a computer in your healthcare profession, you should have it password protected so that others cannot view the records. Only the medical office manager should have the passwords of all computers, and this information must be kept in a secure location.

Scenario 5 is a more common problem than you might think. Many medical offices store patient records within the office/reception area where they can be easily accessed. By not locking these records in a separate area after office hours, there is a chance that workers such as Mr. McMurray could help themselves to reading records. Medical records should always be locked when office employees are not around to protect them. Remember, the more people who handle a medical record, the more chances there are for confidential information to be leaked.

THE HEALTH INSURANCE PORTABILITY AND ACCOUNTABILITY ACT

The Health Insurance Portability and Accountability Act (HIPAA) was signed into law in 1996 under the William Jefferson Clinton administration. This federal law was enacted to address privacy issues and continuation of health insurance coverage in health care. This important legislation gives the patient more control over personal medical information and how it is used or released.

Five different forms are required to protect patient information:

1. The privacy notice
2. The signature of patient indicating that he or she received the privacy notice
3. The patient's permission to provide his or her medical information to other people (such as a relative) or entities (such as an insurance company)
4. A trading partner agreement specifying the parties involved (i.e., physician and patient)
5. A contractual statement between the physician or facility and the patient

The original intent of HIPAA was twofold (Quan, 2007). The first aim was to improve conditions when individuals change health insurance programs, including portability. **Portability** means that no lapse of healthcare coverage occurs when a person changes from one job to another, even when insurance carriers change.

The second aim was to make sure that as long as there is no lapse of coverage, preexisting conditions are covered. **Preexisting conditions** are ailments or diseases that the patient has before health insurance coverage begins. Preexisting conditions often limit healthcare coverage, and this component was designed to help the patient get coverage needed to receive medical care.

Before the HIPAA laws were enacted, a person moving from one job to another had to go for a period of time with no healthcare insurance. This might happen because there was a gap between the two jobs and/or because the new insurance might take a few months to take effect. The preexisting allowance in the law permits continuous coverage through the **Consolidated Omnibus Budget Reconciliation Act (COBRA)**, which is discussed later.

These two factors protect a person's health insurance coverage. Though preventing loss of coverage and protecting individuals with preexisting conditions were the two initial motivators for the HIPAA legislation, Congress decided to also incorporate other factors. The "add-ons" in the final HIPAA legislation include protection of private medical information, standardization and simplification of forms, and strategies to prevent fraud, waste, and abuse.

Acting upon the legislation of the Clinton administration, the George Herbert Walker Bush administration and Congress chose to introduce the law in three phases:

1. Implementation of federal privacy regulations
2. Implementation of insurance claims
3. Implementation of a clearinghouse of electronic medical claims

Though HIPAA was written into law in 1996, phases concerning insurance and clearinghouse implementation did not take effect until 2002, and the phase concerning federal privacy legislation did not take effect until 2003. These delays, some say, were due to complications in implementation, and had to be addressed to make the legislation practical. In other words, it was unclear whether the bill, in its original form, would be practical to carry out.

Knowing that as a healthcare professional you will have this enormous responsibility, it is important for you to pay special attention to the contents of this chapter as well as the information provided in the *Accountability: The Medical Record* chapter. The question you must continually ask yourself is, "How can I achieve confidentiality for the sake of the patient?" **(Figure 4-3)**.

The two primary answers to this question are *professional silence* and *secure data management*. More specifically, your best defense against violating confidentiality is to know the HIPAA laws and how they pertain to patients.

Access to a patient's medical record does not give automatic permission to view the record. For example, suppose you work in an outpatient clinic as a receptionist. Your work area is where the medical records are stored. Just because you *could* pull any of the records and read them, does not mean that you should. Most likely, as a medical receptionist, your job does not require you to work with patient records. Therefore, you "have no business" opening and reading a patient's medical record. If you do not need to read the record to assist in serving the patient, you should not access it at all. This is sometimes called the "need to know" clause in HIPAA legislation.

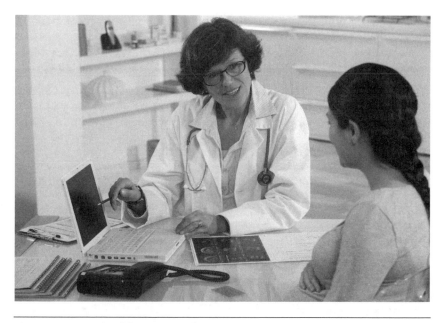

Figure 4-3 As a healthcare provider, you must always consider how to best protect your patient's medical information.

There are five primary components of the HIPAA law:

1. Title l: Insurance Portability
2. Title II: Administrative Simplification
3. Title III: Medical Savings and Tax Deduction
4. Title IV: Group Health Plan Provisions
5. Title V: Revenue Offset Provisions

The Consolidated Omnibus Budget Reconciliation Act

The Consolidated Omnibus Budget Reconciliation Act of 1985 (COBRA) was a forerunner to HIPAA. In essence, COBRA mandates that those businesses with 20 employees or more must provide employees who leave that business extended health insurance for up to 18 months. This insurance can be at the expense of the company but usually is paid for by the employee. Many employees are

Table 4-1 An Example of How COBRA Can Affect Healthcare Insurance

September 15, 2011	September 16, 2011	March 12, 2012	March 14, 2012
The ACME Corporation lays off 200 of its 1,200 workers due to economic conditions. Nikita Washington is one of those workers. She decides to purchase the health insurance from ACME through COBRA until she gets a new job and new health insurance coverage.	Nikita begins paying ACME $385 per month to continue her health insurance. This coverage was free when she worked for ACME.	Nikita is hired by the RalStar Company. Her insurance with RalStar begins immediately. She no longer has to pay ACME for health insurance coverage.	Nikita would have lost her COBRA coverage on this date, so she is fortunate to have gotten a new job when she did.

provided health insurance free of charge through the company. If the employee leaves that place of employment, he or she may then decide to purchase the coverage until other coverage takes effect **(Table 4-1)**. This continuity of coverage could be the difference, for example, between paying $10 for a medication under coverage and paying $200 without coverage.

The Privacy Rule

The **Privacy Rule** went into effect in 2001 and was fully implemented in 2003. It is the portion of HIPAA that refers to personal data (past, present, and future), otherwise known as **protected health information (PHI)**. PHI is specific medical information pertaining to the patient, such as name, date of birth, and social security number. One crucial treatment of PHI is that concerning the patient and health insurance companies, also known as vendors. Health insurance companies may obtain medical information about a patient, but only if the patient signs a release of information. PHI can come in three primary forms: written, electronic, and even oral. There are some exceptions to PHI, including suspected abuse (including elder, child, and spousal abuse), medical research, and certain contagious diseases. These exceptions vary from state to state according to state law.

PHI does have its limitations. It does not include information a person shares with law enforcement officials, bankers or creditors, insurance representatives, school teachers or administrators, or employers. Although it is not legally mandated, it would be professionally sound and ethical conduct for all professionals to protect the personal information of any client. This lack of protection might prompt many people to limit their sharing of confidential health information to the healthcare provider, who is legally obligated to keep medical information in the strictest of confidence. Failure to do so could result in the healthcare professional being punished, ranging from a fine to imprisonment. Keep in mind that health information includes pharmacy records and mental health records and is not limited to the confines of a hospital or physician's office.

Exceptions to HIPAA (Bureau, 2004)

You might expect a law as strong as HIPAA to cover everything, but that is not the case. HIPAA does not cover the following:

- Financial documents (credit information, banking records)
- Information as maintained by the Central Intelligence Agency (CIA), as outlined in the Privacy Act of 1974 (U.S. Department of Justice, 2003)
- Educational records (including vaccinations and other information)
- Subpoenas for medical records needed in court cases
- The electronic database files of private companies
- Employment records, including any employer-sponsored health program in which you may participate or information needed by your employer for the Family and Medical Leave Act (FMLA) (It is important to also know that if a company is self-insured for medical coverage of employees, the handling of insurance claims and other health-related information *is* covered by HIPAA.)

It would seem that any personal record would be covered, but often information is covered by other laws such as the FMLA and the Gramm-Leach-Bliley Act (GLB). For more information on medical information, safety records, and/or family and medical leave records, visit the U.S. Department of Labor website at http://www.dol.gov.

Healthcare Integrity and Protection Data Bank

The **Healthcare Integrity and Protection Data Bank (HIPDB)** was established under HIPAA and became fully operational in 2000. This national data bank was an aggressive move to prevent fraudulent and/or abusive healthcare practitioners and suppliers from being able to practice. Areas being monitored, as outlined in the Social Security Act, include:

- Licensure and certification actions
- Exclusion from participation in federal and state healthcare programs (e.g., Medicare)
- Civil judgments related to health care
- Criminal convictions
- Revocation or suspension of lab certification

Centralized data banks such as the HIPDB were designed to improve not just the ethical standards and practices of the healthcare industry, but also to provide a go-to place to prevent unethical persons from being allowed to serve patients. Think of the HIPDB, in some ways, as a "Better Business Bureau of Healthcare".

Release of Information

A patient's medical information is protected under HIPAA laws, and there are specific rules about who can have access to that information. When a patient is under the care of a physician, for example, that patient's medical information cannot be discussed with anyone else unless the patient so allows it. A **release of information** form is a document that allows the healthcare provider to share certain information—not necessarily the whole record **(Figure 4-4)**.

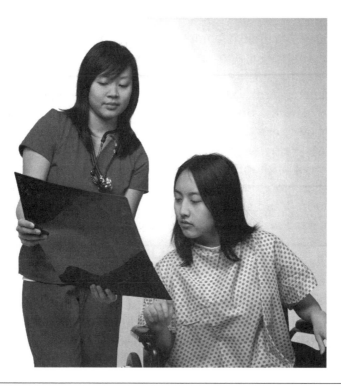

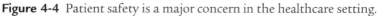

Figure 4-4 Patient safety is a major concern in the healthcare setting.

Case Study: Releasing Medical Information

Suppose you work in a factory where you do heavy lifting on a daily basis. It is Wednesday and you have been having headaches and shooting pains in your back since Monday morning. With the permission of your supervisor, Janet Reid, you leave work and go to your family physician, Dr. Carlos Mendez. After a thorough examination, it is revealed that you are having complex migraine headaches and are ordered to bed rest for 2 days with a new medication. You call in to work to let Ms. Reid know that you have a physician's excuse and will return to work on

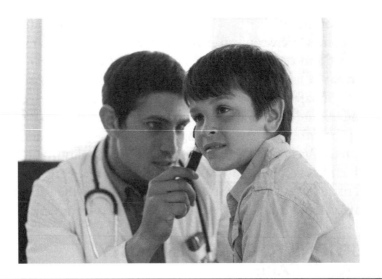

Figure 4-5 Healthcare professionals are legally required to report suspected child abuse.

Every 10 seconds in America, a report is made concerning the mal-treatment of a child. Considering that many incidents of child abuse go unreported, it is undeniable that child abuse is a major concern. The following professionals are legally required to report suspected child abuse (Newton, 2001):

- Physicians
- Nurses
- Dentists
- Mental health professionals
- Social workers
- Teachers
- Day care workers
- Law enforcement personnel

In some states, clergy, foster parents, attorneys, and camp coun-selors also are required to report abuse. In 18 states, *any person* who suspects abuse is required to report it.

When a healthcare professional recognizes any sign of abuse (including suspect bruises or fractures, and/or the child being with-drawn or upset), he or she is legally obligated to report to the suspi-cions to the county's Department of Human Services and the police department. Reports can also be made to the 24-hour Child Abuse National Hotline: 1-800-4-A-CHILD (1-800-252-2873). As a healthcare professional, this phone number should be in your phone list.

Elder Abuse

Like child abuse, elder abuse occurs in a specific age group and many cases go unreported. Though legal definitions vary from state to state (including the age, which ranges from 50 years upward), a general definition could be "any harmful treatment of an elderly person." Harmful treatment can include physical, emotional, or sexual abuse; neglect; financial exploitation; and self-abuse.

According to the National Research Council Panel to Review Risk and Prevalence of Elder Abuse and Neglect (2003), "It has been estimated that between 1 and 2 million Americans 65 years or older have been injured, exploited, or otherwise mistreated by someone on whom they depended for care or protection." Healthcare professionals should always report any suspected cases of elder abuse, including self-inflicted abuse **(Figure 4-6)**. If a healthcare professional suspects

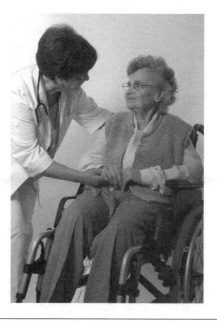

Figure 4-6 Healthcare professionals are legally required to report suspected elder abuse.

elder abuse, he or she should immediately contact the local police department and the local Department of Human Services. In 16 states, reporting is mandated. In those states, not reporting could result in criminal charges, just as in instances of not reporting child abuse.

Mental Health Patients Who Might Pose a Threat

Mental illness affects at least one in five Americans. Just like children and senior citizens, mental health patients are part of a specific vulnerable population. Psychiatrists and psychologists may seem to be the professionals who would most frequently encounter this situation, but, in fact, any healthcare professional may serve a patient with mental illness because many of these individuals are not institutionalized. Any healthcare professional has a legal and ethical obligation to report even a suspicion of a mental patient in self-harm or one who is harming others.

Matters of the Greater Good

Though confidentiality is decidedly one of the highest priorities in health care, there are times when the best interest of the public outweighs the protection of a patient's private medical information.

Case Study: William Gladstone

William Gladstone works at the Superior Furniture Company, which employs 2,500 people in Northern Texas. Superior just sponsored a company picnic where 4,210 employees and their family members attended. William attended the picnic with his family. After the picnic, the Gladstones went home, commenting on the good time they had. About an hour after returning home, William began feeling nauseous and vomited several times. He had strong stomach cramps and also developed a fever with chills. When the pain became unbearable, William's wife took him to the emergency room of the local community hospital. After a thorough examination and some diagnostic tests, it was concluded that William had food poisoning, and after some investigation, it was discovered that the potato salad at the picnic had been outside in the heat for over 2 hours and had spoiled, causing food poisoning.

The attending physician took William's information, letting him know that he was going to contact the local health department and also Superior to let them know. It turned out that more than 200 people who ate the potato salad contracted food poisoning. By reporting William's food poisoning, others were alerted so they could seek medical treatment. William's name was not given, but to serve the greater good (the general public), food poisoning was reported and eventually that information helped others. The case of William Gladstone might not be considered as urgent and as life threatening as other conditions, such as the spread of Anthrax, but it could have ended in tragedy all the same.

Alerting the public to a potential danger can help ensure their safety. In the William Gladstone case study, reporting the botulism (food poisoning) certainly helped those who attended the picnic and could have saved lives. Normally a patient's medical information is kept in total confidence, but sometimes the benefits to the general public warrant reporting.

PUTTING IT ALL TOGETHER

No matter how you slice it, confidentiality is a right of every patient in the United States. The patient has a say in how his or her medical information is shared, with a few exceptions. These exceptions are covered by federal laws, including the Privacy Act of 1974 and HIPAA.

As a healthcare professional, it is your responsibility to protect patient information. Experience and practice will help you reach the highest standards in this regard. Whether you are in your place of employment or out in public, your knowledge of patients' medical information should never be shared with others, generally speaking.

CHAPTER CHECKUP

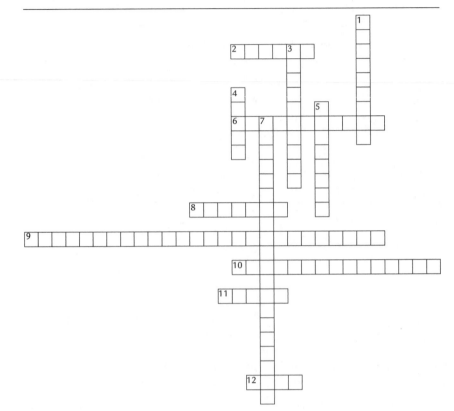

Crossword Puzzle

Across

2. To violate.
6. No lapse of healthcare coverage.
8. PHI can come in three forms: oral, electronic, and _____.
9. Specific medical information of the patient. (3 words)
10. Keeping information private.
11. You may get information on medical information, safety records, and/or family and medical leave records from the Department of _____.

12. Name of the president who signed into law the Privacy Act of 1974.

Down

1. HIPAA does not cover financial _____.
3. One exception to confidentiality of medical information. (2 words)
4. Important legislation that gives the patient more control over personal medical information and how it is used or released.
5. The number of states that have a law that any person who suspects abuse is required to report it.
7. A document that allows the healthcare provider to share certain information. (3 words)

REFERENCES

Department of Health and Human Services. (1999). Annual prevalence of mental/addictive disorders for children in mental health: A report of the Surgeon General, *U.S. Department of Health and Human Services, Substance Abuse and Mental Health Services Administration, with NIH.* Washington, DC: U.S. Government Printing Office.

HIV/AIDS Bureau. (2004, April). Protecting health information privacy and complying with federal regulations: A resource guide for HIV services providers and the Health Resources and Services Administration's HIV/AIDS Bureau Staff. Retrieved from ftp://ftp.hrsa.gov/hab/hipaa04.pdf

National Research Council Panel to Review Risk and Prevalence of Elder Abuse and Neglect. (2003). Elder mistreatment: Abuse, neglect and exploitation in an aging America. Washington, DC.

Newton, C. J. (2001, April). Child abuse: An overview. *Mental Health Journal.* Retrieved from http://www.findcounseling.com/journal/child-abuse/child-abuse-laws.html

Quan K. (2007, November 19). Confidentiality in health care: Health care professionals must learn the rules of confidentiality. Retrieved from http://suite101.com/article/confidentiality-in-health-care-a3593

U.S. Department of Health and Human Services. (n.d.). Health Information Privacy. Retrieved from http://www.hhs.gov/ocr/privacy/psa/understanding/index.html

U.S. Department of Justice. (2003). The Privacy Act of 1974, section 552a. Retrieved from http://www.justice.gov/opcl/privstat.htm

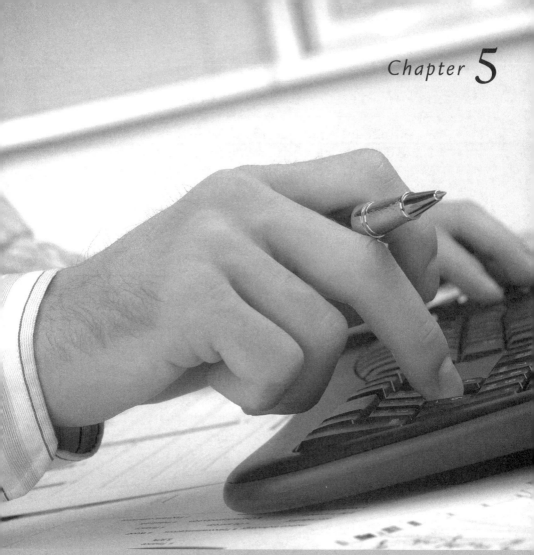

Chapter 5

Ethics and the Workplace

It takes less time to do a thing right than to explain why you did it wrong.

—Henry Wadsworth Longfellow

IN THIS CHAPTER, YOU WILL LEARN ABOUT:

- Laws surrounding employment in health care
- What to do if you are a victim of discrimination
- How to find the code of ethics related to your profession
- Medical practice acts
- Ethical issues surrounding the healthcare workplace
- How to report an ethics violation
- The progressive discipline technique

KEY TERMS

Age Discrimination in Employment Act
Americans With Disabilities Act (ADA)
Civil Rights Act
Equal Employment Opportunity Commission (EEOC)
Equal Pay Act
Fair Labor Standards Act (FLSA)

Family and Medical Leave Act
Medical practice acts
Occupational Safety and Health Act
Patient Protection and Affordable Care Act
Pregnancy Discrimination Act
Progressive discipline model
Rehabilitation Act

For Your Consideration

Health care is a business. Most people might choose to go into health care because of a desire to help others and contribute to society, but first and foremost, it is still a business. Is it possible to find a balance between running a successful business and helping society? Most healthcare professions have a code of ethics that attempts to find that balance. Understanding the laws and ethical principles that surround the healthcare environment is a wonderful place to start.

WORKPLACE LAWS AND HEALTHCARE PROFESSIONALS

After obtaining a degree in health care, Tania begins searching for employment. She is recently married and expecting her first child. She hopes to find a job with flexible hours and decent benefits. She is concerned that employers will not consider giving her a job because she is pregnant or that she will lose her job when she takes time off after her baby is born. Tania remembers learning something about these topics in one of the first classes she took toward her degree, so she sends her professor an e-mail expressing her concerns. The professor responds with a reminder of some of the laws related to employment, as well as a helpful chart of questions that employers are legally allowed to ask during an interview and questions that they should not ask.

There are several federal laws that employers must follow. The **Fair Labor Standards Act (FLSA)** of 1938 sets minimum wage limits, regulates overtime pay standards, and establishes guidelines for youth employment **(Figure 5-1)**. All employers must comply with the FLSA,

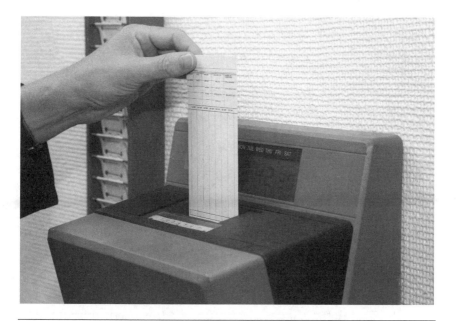

Figure 5-1 The Fair Labor Standards Act of 1938 addresses such employment issues as minimum wage, overtime, and youth employment.

except small, independently owned construction, retail, and service businesses. Certain provisions under this act specifically apply to healthcare professionals (United States Department of Labor, 2010).

- The **Equal Pay Act** prohibits sex-based wage differences between men and women employed in the same establishment who perform jobs that require equal skill, effort, and responsibility and that are performed under similar working conditions. This act does not mean that men and women will always receive the same pay, because other factors also help determine an employee's pay rate (e.g., years on the job, education).
- The **Family and Medical Leave Act** requires employers, given qualifying circumstances, to allow employees up to 12 weeks of unpaid job-protected leave each year after at least 1 year of employment that includes at least 1,250 hours of work. The 12 weeks can include sick leave and vacation time already provided by the employer; it does not have to be in addition to it. An employee can request leave for the birth and care of an infant; adopting or accepting a foster child; care of a sick child, spouse, or parent; or the employee's serious health condition.
- The newest of the legislations discussed here is the **Patient Protection and Affordable Care Act** (signed into law in March 2010), which includes a requirement that employees provide reasonable break time for new mothers to pump breast milk. This requirement lasts for 1 year after the birth of a child and includes an appropriate setting for expressing the milk, which excludes bathrooms.

All of these laws are overseen and enforced by the Wage and Hour Division of the U.S. Department of Labor, except for the Equal Pay Act. While the Equal Pay Act is a provision of the Fair Labor Standards Act (FLSA), it is actually overseen by the **Equal Employment Opportunity Commission (EEOC)**. The EEOC also oversees several other laws important to healthcare professionals (United States Equal Employment Opportunity Commission, n.d.):

- The **Civil Rights Act** of 1964 prohibits the discrimination of anyone based on sex and race during the hiring, promoting, and firing processes. Title VII of this act changes the wording to prohibit employment discrimination on the basis of race, color, religion, sex, or national origin (National Archives, n.d.).

- The **Age Discrimination in Employment Act** of 1967 prohibits employment discrimination against individuals 40 years of age or older.
- The **Rehabilitation Act** of 1973 requires that employees not discriminate against qualified individuals based on disability. This means that if a disabled individual is able to perform the job duties required with minimal accommodations from the employer, he or she is protected from discrimination. This act only applies to organizations receiving financial assistance from the federal government (e.g., Medicaid reimbursement to a hospital) (United States Department of Health and Human Services, 2006).
- The **Pregnancy Discrimination Act of 1978** amends Title VII of the Civil Rights Act. This act makes it illegal for an employer to refuse to hire a woman because she is pregnant. It also prohibits firing a woman who is pregnant simply because she is pregnant or forcing her to go on maternity leave.
- The **Americans With Disabilities Act (ADA)** of 1992 prohibits discrimination of individuals with physical or mental disabilities **(Figure 5-2)**. It extends the Rehabilitation Act of 1973 to all employers with at least 15 employees. Any substantial physical or mental impairment that limits at least one significant life activity (e.g., walking, cognition, breathing, communication, seeing) is considered a disability. This act includes individuals with AIDS and HIV infections. It also applies to past disabilities and association with someone who is disabled. For example, if your spouse has HIV, an employer cannot refuse to hire you for fear that your spouse will have expensive health insurance premiums. The ADA covers some cases of rehabilitated drug addicts and alcoholics, as well as some instances of obesity. Employers who hire someone with a disability might be required to make minor modification to the work environment, such as ramps or handicapped-accessible bathrooms. If the employer can prove that the expense of such accommodations would cause an undue hardship on the business,

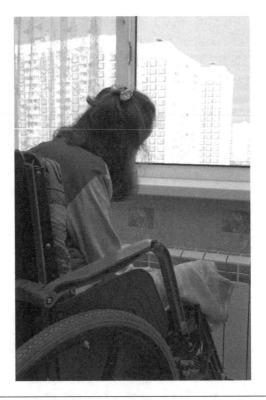

Figure 5-2 The disabled citizen is protected under the Americans With Disabilities Act, which prohibits discrimination of individuals with physical or mental disabilities.

the employer can often legally refuse to hire the individual. In addition, the person with a disability would need to be able to perform specific job functions similar to other employees, and job offers can be contingent on a medical exam, but only if the exam is required of all potential employees.

During the interview process, it is not necessarily illegal to ask certain questions, but the Equal Employment and Opportunity Commission (EEOC) has strict guidelines that employers should follow. In general, questions should not be discriminatory in nature. It is fine for future employees to volunteer information on age, marital status, and religion, for example, but employers should not ask those types of questions. **Table 5-1** lists examples of questions that should and should not be asked during an interview.

Table 5-1 Questions That Should and Should Not Be Asked During an Interview

Topic	Legitimate Questions	Illegitimate Questions
Citizenship	• Are you authorized to work in the United States? • In which languages do you consider yourself fluent?	• Are you a U.S. citizen? • Where were you or your parents born? • What do you consider to be your native language?
Age	• Are you at least 18 years old?	• How old are you? • When did you graduate from high school? • What is your date of birth?
Family status	• Would you be willing to relocate if necessary? • Would you be available to travel as needed for this job? • Would you be available to work overtime as necessary?	• Are you married? • Who lives in your house? • Do you plan to have a family? When? • How many children do you have? • What type of child care do you use?
Affiliations	• What professional or trade organizations related to this job do you have membership in?	• What clubs or social organizations do you have membership in?
Disabilities	• Are you able to perform all the essential duties required of this job? • Can you demonstrate how you would perform (specific job duty required)?	• Do you have any disabilities? • Have you had any recent or past illnesses or operations? • When was your last physical exam? • How is the health of your family members? • When/how did you lose your (function such as eyesight or hearing)?
Criminal record	• Have you ever been convicted of (a crime that is reasonably related to job duties or honesty)?	• Have you ever been arrested?
Military history	• In what branch of the military did you serve?	• Were you honorably discharged from the military?

In our scenario at the beginning of this chapter, Tania feels much more secure after learning about the laws that protect her rights. She interviews for a few positions and is offered a job with some flexibility and good benefits. She understands that the Family Medical Leave Act will not apply to her because she will not have had her job for at least 1 year before her child is born. However, she is comfortable with her employer and is able to compromise the use of her vacation and sick leave to accommodate her maternity leave.

Fortunately, Tania does not feel any discrimination from her employer, but what if an employee does feel that he or she has been a victim of discrimination? According to the Equal Employment Opportunity Commission (EEOC), any suspected cases of discrimination may be filed in person, by mail, or by phone at the nearest EEOC office. There are specific guidelines for filing charges based on the offense. Generally, an individual has 180 days to file a complaint for violations of the Civil Rights Act, the Americans With Disabilities Act, or the Age Discrimination Act. If the EEOC determines that discrimination has occurred, it will first contact the employer and attempt to conciliate. Conciliation might involve asking the company to hire or rehire, promote, or award back pay to the victim of discrimination. The employer might also be fined and forced to make policy changes. If this attempt at conciliation fails, the EEOC will file a lawsuit on the victim's behalf. It is also possible for the victim to hire a private lawyer and sue the employer at his or her own expense (United States Equal Employment Opportunity Commission, 1997).

Case in Point: Cheryl Hall

In April 2003, Cheryl Hall was working as a sales secretary for a Chicago-based company. She requested and was given time off to undergo in vitro fertilization. The first treatment was unsuccessful and resulted in 20 days of missed work. Ms. Hall requested another leave of absence in July, 2003, for a second in vitro fertilization treatment. At the same time, the Chicago-based company was consolidating with another company, which required the downsizing of employees. This downsizing included the reduction of sales secretaries from two to one. Ms. Hall was informed of her termination at the end of July, and her supervisor informed her that it was probably for the best, due to her health status.

After her termination, Ms. Hall filed a complaint with the EEOC within the appropriate time period. The EEOC declined to intervene, but did provide a Notice of Right to Sue. Ms. Hall filed an action against the company (Nalco) alleging sexual discrimination based on Title VII of the Civil Rights Act of 1964. Her complaint included discrimination of a pro-tected class: a female with the pregnancy-related condition of infertility. The district court disagreed and ruled in favor of Nalco. The basis of their decision was that both men and women can suffer from infertility. On appeal, the U.S. Court of Appeals for the Seventh Circuit reversed the decision. They agreed that infertility can affect both sexes, but only women take time off for in vitro fertilization treatments. Ms. Hall's case was sent back to trial court (Hall v. Nalco Company, 534 F3d 644, 2008).

Tania, the subject of our case study, and her husband decide to move to a new state to be closer to family. They both quit their jobs and plan to find new jobs after the move. Tania remembers that she has certain rights related to the benefits package provided by her former employer. She contacts her employer to learn more about these benefits. Known as COBRA, the Consolidated Omnibus Budget Reconciliation Act of 1985 refers to an employee's right to purchase healthcare benefits available from his or her employer for a certain length of time. The employee must pay the same premium as the employer but cannot be denied benefits. This law is helpful to employ-ees who are changing jobs because it prevents future healthcare insurers from refusing to provide coverage for preexisting conditions (United States Department of Labor, n.d.).

One final law that is important for healthcare professionals is the **Occupational Safety and Health Act**, which is administered by the Occupational Safety and Health Administration (OSHA). OSHA is responsible for regulating the safety and health conditions of most private and public work environments. Employers are responsible for maintaining a safe work environment for employees and patrons. In addition, OSHA has laws specific to the healthcare industry. According to OSHA's website, more workers are injured in healthcare and social services industries than in any other industry **(Figure 5-3)**. Risks for injuries include:

- Exposure to bloodborne pathogens, biologic hazards, chemicals, and drugs
- Ergonomic hazards from lifting and repetitious tasks

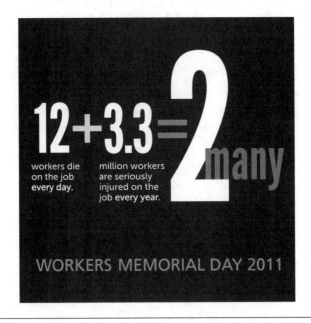

Figure 5-3 This visual was used in a 2011 OSHA campaign to illustrate the injuries and lives lost on the job daily.

Source: Solis, S. H. (2011, April 28). One is Too Many. Retrieved April 10, 2012, from (Work in Progress) The Official Blog of the U.S. Department of Labor: http://social.dol.gov/blog/one-is-too-many/

- Workplace violence
- Laboratory hazards
- Exposure to radioactive materials, including x-rays (United States Department of Labor, n.d.).

Healthcare professionals should be aware of potential risks to their health and safety. It is the employer's responsibility to raise awareness of these risks, as well as to train employees in safe practices, such as proper disposal of hazardous waste and proper lifting techniques. Complying with OSHA regulations requires up-to-date knowledge of any changes. For example, while bed rails used to be common in most healthcare facilities to protect patients, they have been replaced with lowered beds and floor mats to avoid claims of false imprisonment.

Case in Point: Acadia Hospital

In 2010, OSHA cited Acadia Hospital in Bangor, Maine, for failing to provide adequate safeguards against workplace violence. The inspection was prompted by complaints from employees at the facility. During the investigation, OSHA found at least 115 instances between 2008 and 2010 of assault from violent patients against employees in the psychiatric hospital and clinic. OSHA cited the facility for failure to provide a workplace free from recognized hazards likely to cause death or serious injury. The facility was charged nearly $12,000 in combined fines and given several suggestions on policies to implement (United States Department of Labor, 2011).

THE HEALTHCARE TEAM—WHAT IS YOUR ROLE?

Starting a job in health care can be overwhelming. There are many different types of professionals in health care, and they interact in various ways. For example, in a long-term care facility, speech therapists might work closely with dieticians, certified nursing assistants, registered nurses, occupational therapists, physical therapists, and doctors. All of these professionals have different roles and responsibilities, known as scope of practice. In an effort to work together as a team, it is necessary to understand the general scope of practice of each profession. **Table 5-2** lists various healthcare professions and their general scope of practice.

It is important to be familiar with the various roles in health care, not only for yourself but for patients as well. If a patient has a specific

Table 5-2 Various Healthcare Professions and Their General Scope of Practice

Profession	General Scope of Practice
Audiologist	Diagnoses and treats hearing and balance disorders.
Dental hygienist	Provides preventive dental care, such as cleaning and x-rays. Is overseen by a dentist, and assists the dentist with procedures.
Dentist	Prevents and treats disorders of the oral cavity.
Dietician	Provides expertise in food and nutrition. Assists patients in diet planning.
Doctor/physician	Focuses on diagnosis and treatment of illnesses and injuries. There are various specialties in this field.
Emergency medical technician (EMT)	Provides care for the sick or injured in emergency settings.
Fitness trainer	Provides guidance toward health and wellness through exercise.
Healthcare administrator/manager	Manages healthcare facilities.
Health information technologist	Organizes and manages health information data.
Massage therapist	Treats body disorders through manipulation of soft tissue.
Medical assistant	Performs clinical and administrative tasks to assist physicians.
Medical office manager	Manages the operation of the medical office.
Medical transcriptionist	Converts physician dictations into text format.
Nurse (LPN/LVN, CAN, RN)	Performs various duties, depending on degree and state regulations. All provide health-related care for patients and families.

Table 5-2 Various Healthcare Professions and Their General Scope
of Practice (*continued*)

Profession	General Scope of Practice
Occupational therapist	Provides therapy related to daily tasks, with a focus on fine-motor skills.
Pharmacist	Dispenses medications prescribed by healthcare professionals.
Pharmacy technician	Performs pharmacy-related duties under the supervision of a pharmacist.
Physical therapist	Provides therapy to regain skills after injury or illness, with a focus on large-motor skills.
Respiratory therapist	Provides care for patients who have trouble breathing.
Speech therapist	Provides therapy to patients with speech, language, cognitive, or swallowing disorders.

need that is outside of your scope of practice, you should take time to explain this to the patient and direct him or her to the appropriate professional. Knowing which healthcare professional can best serve his or her needs can help alleviate the patient's anxiety and give him or her knowledge to promote self-advocacy in the future.

Knowing the various roles of healthcare professionals can help overall relations in the workplace. For example, if a dietician repeatedly asks a certified nursing assistant (CNA) for a patient's medication list, it might frustrate the CNA to have to explain that most states do not allow CNAs to distribute medications and that this task falls under the registered nurse's scope of practice. Awareness of job duties helps to streamline the multiple tasks that healthcare professionals are faced with on a daily basis.

Working in a healthcare environment also requires the ability to work well with a variety of different people. Certain standards of professionalism must be observed in an effort to provide a safe environment for patients. These standards include, but are not limited to:

- Keeping up to date with training and education in your field
- Addressing the health needs of society
- Complying with laws and regulations governing your field

- Acting in a trustworthy manner toward patients, employers, and fellow employees
- Completing job tasks in a prompt and dependable manner

In health care, as in most professions, you might run into coworkers and employers who do not share your personal values or point of view. In these cases, it is important to remember that we come from diverse backgrounds. If healthcare professionals strive to act as professionals in the healthcare setting, most issues will be avoided. When conflicts do arise, it is best to first approach the fellow healthcare professional in a calm manner. If that is not successful, you may need to enlist the help of a supervisor. If the conflict persists, but is truly just a conflict of personal values, the healthcare professional will have to decide whether the working environment is still tolerable or whether he or she might need to consider seeking employment elsewhere. The important thing to remember is that any personal conflicts between employees (or employer and employee) need to be settled in a manner that does not involve or disrupt patient care. If it does, it might become an ethical violation.

All healthcare professionals must follow the code of ethics related to their profession. It is simple to find the code of ethics for your professional organization by searching on the internet. Nearly all professional organizations have websites dedicated to professionals and the public. These websites provide information on licensure, certification, careers, continuing education, and professional codes of ethics. See the box titled "Professional Association of Health Office Management (PAHCOM): Code of Ethics (2012)" for a typical code of ethics for a healthcare profession. **Table 5-3** provides a list of common healthcare professions and their professional organizations.

Professional Association of Health Care Office Management (PAHCOM): Code of Ethics (2012)

1. *PAHCOM* members shall be dedicated to providing the highest standard of managerial services to employers, employees, and patients, showing compassion and respect for human dignity.

2. *PAHCOM* members shall maintain the highest standard of professional conduct.
3. *PAHCOM* members shall respect the rights of patients, employers, and employees, and within the constraints of the law, maintain the confidentiality of all privileged information.
4. *PAHCOM* members shall use only legal and ethical means in all professional dealings, and shall refuse to cooperate with, or condone by silence, the actions of those who engage in fraudulent, deceptive, or illegal acts.
5. *PAHCOM* members shall respect the laws and regulations of the land, and the bylaws of the Association, and recognize a responsibility to seek to change those laws which are contrary to the best interest of patients, employers, employees, and other Association members.
6. *PAHCOM* members shall pursue excellence through continuing education in all areas applicable to the management of the medical office.
7. *PAHCOM* members shall strive to maintain and enhance the dignity, status, competence, and standards of medical office management and its practitioners.
8. *PAHCOM* members shall use every opportunity, including participation in local health care associations, to promote and improve public understanding and enhancement of the status of the profession.
9. *PAHCOM* members shall respect the integrity and protect the welfare of employers, employees, and patients.
10. *PAHCOM* members do not exploit professional relationships with patients, employees, or employers for personal gain. Nor do they condone or engage in sexual harassment or discriminatory hiring and supervisory practices.

Courtesy of: Professional Association of Health Care Office Management.

Table 5-3 Common Healthcare Professions and Their Professional
Organizations

Profession	Organization
Audiologist	American Academy of Audiology
Dietician	American Dietetic Association
Health information technologist	American Health Information Management Association
Healthcare administrator	American Association of Healthcare Administrative Management
	Association for Healthcare Administrative Professionals
	Health Care Administrators Association
Massage therapist	American Massage Therapy Association
Medical assistant	American Association of Medical Assistants
Medical office manager	Professional Association of Health Care Office Management
Medical transcriptionist	Association for Healthcare Documentation Integrity
Nurse	American Nurses Association
Occupational therapist	American Occupational Therapy Association
Physical therapist	American Physical Therapy Association
Physician	American Medical Association
	American Osteopathic Association
Speech therapist	American Speech, Language, and Hearing Association

In addition to professional organizations, most states have laws
related to licensure and certification. These **medical practice acts** vary
from state to state and serve to govern the practice of medicine. Once a
healthcare professional obtains a degree, he or she will need to obtain a
license or certificate from the state in which he or she wishes to obtain
a job. Information on licensure and certification can be found through
the websites of the organizations listed in Table 5-3. If a healthcare
professional moves to a new state, he or she will be required to apply
for a new license or certificate to legally practice in that state.

> ## Case Study: Reporting Professional Misconduct
>
> After working at a local hospital for several years, Percy was offered a promotion to work as a nurse in the rehabilitation department. When he started his job, he noticed that several nurses seemed relieved to have a male in the department. After a few days on the job, Percy was surprised to learn that the rehabilitation doctor made rude comments and occasionally groped the female nurses. Percy spoke to his fellow nurses and learned that this had been occurring for several years, but none of the nurses were willing to risk their jobs in order to report the well-respected rehabilitation doctor. Percy decided he would look into reporting the unethical behavior.

What steps should be taken to report an ethics violation? In general, ethical violations should be reported at the place of employment first. If you feel comfortable, it might be beneficial to approach the fellow employee first. Sometimes a coworker is not aware that his or her behavior is unethical and simply needs a reminder. If that is out of your comfort zone, you might consider notifying your supervisor. Most facilities also have an anonymous box to report ethics violations. If your supervisor is the one behaving unethically, it might be necessary to file a complaint at the state medical society or licensing board. Some states allow anonymous complaints to be filed, but certain states (e.g., Texas) no longer allow complaints to be filed anonymously. The purpose is to protect those who file complaints. If the complaints are anonymous, it is not possible for the filer to prove that he or she was discriminated against for filing a complaint. The new policy is to keep the complaints confidential.

Once a complaint is filed, the licensing board completes an investigation, seeking evidence and witnesses, as necessary. After the investigation, the board reviews the findings and determines if there is enough proof to support the claim. If a healthcare professional is found to have committed an ethics violation, there is a risk of civil penalties, as well as the possibility of job loss and loss of license. No criminal charges can be filed for strictly ethical violations. In some cases, the healthcare professional may be required to pay restitution to the affected parties. When making these decisions, the state licensing board will determine whether to suspend or revoke the employee's license. It is up to the employer whether to discipline or terminate the employee. Several options are available to the employer based on the severity of the violation and the number of violations the healthcare professional has had in the past.

An employer that decides to discipline the healthcare professional rather than terminate him or her might use a **progressive discipline model (Figure 5-4)**. The purpose of progressive discipline is to encourage the employee to improve job performance, rather than to punish. These types of models vary, but typically involve the following steps:

1. Provide counseling or a verbal warning.
2. Give a written warning with specific guidelines for improved performance.

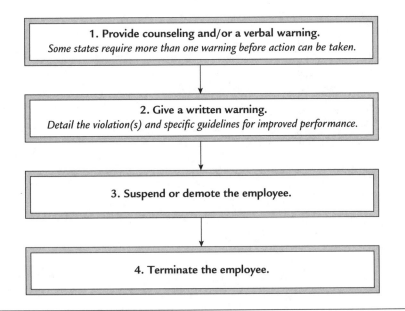

Figure 5-4 The progressive discipline model.

3. Suspend or demote the employee.
4. Terminate the employee.

It should be noted that these types of penalties only apply to healthcare professionals who have committed an ethical violation. Any criminal action would be treated differently. If a healthcare professional commits a crime, the proper authorities should be notified immediately.

As mentioned in our preceding case study, Percy felt that he should file an ethics complaint. He chose to take his complaint to the CEO of the hospital, who dealt with the complaint in an appropriate manner. The CEO interviewed the nursing staff, as well as patients of the doctor. He also visited the rehabilitation wing of the hospital several different times during the week. After gathering evidence, he decided to verbally warn the doctor and provide education on appropriate and ethical behavior. The doctor was reminded that ethical behavior extends to fellow employees, not just patients. Finally, the CEO warned the doctor that he would notify the medical licensing board if any future complaints were received. Some nurses felt that they would prefer to work in a different area of the hospital, and this request was granted. Overall, Percy felt that he made the right decision—for both himself and his fellow employees.

Terminating an employee is not enjoyable, but there are times when it is the most appropriate option. If termination is the chosen action, it must be done fairly and through proper channels. For example, any actions leading up to the termination must be well documented. Specifics must be discussed with the employee including all reasons for termination, steps taken to counsel the employee about the problem, and details about when employment will end.

If you are in a supervisory role, always be sure that an employee understands his or her role in the workplace and that clear expectations are given. Also, a systematic plan for evaluation (annually, for example) helps keep staff in line with standards and performance measures. A thorough interview before hiring (or more than one) is always in order, though you cannot predict trouble in the future.

Knowing and understanding the legal and ethical issues surrounding the healthcare environment is crucial in running a successful healthcare business. Laws do not always stay the same, so it is necessary to stay up to date on new laws or any changes to existing laws. In general, any new laws related to health care provide time for employees and employers to make necessary changes, and the penalties for failing to comply with laws make it worth the time to stay informed. Ethical policies, on the other hand, stay fairly consistent. Nonetheless, as new generations of healthcare employees enter the workforce, it might be necessary to review policies with staff.

PUTTING IT ALL TOGETHER

In a perfect world, there would be no need for laws or law enforcement, but since it is not a perfect world, we should be thankful for laws that protect us. Laws concerning the healthcare industry are many, and though you, the healthcare professional, do not have to know every detail of each one, you should know the most prominent laws in your state of practice relating to the healthcare industry. As both a healthcare professional and a healthcare consumer, it is to your advantage to keep updated on these laws.

CHAPTER CHECKUP

Fill-in-the-Blank

1. The _____ _____ _____ _____ sets minimum wage limits, regulates overtime pay standards, and establishes guidelines for youth employment.
2. The _____ _____ _____ _____ _____ prohibits employment discrimination against individuals 40 years of age or older.
3. OSHA is responsible for regulating the _____ and _____ _____ conditions of most private and public work environments.
4. All healthcare professionals must follow the _____ _____ _____ related to their profession.
5. _____ _____ _____ vary from state to state and serve to govern the practice of medicine.

True/False

1. The Family and Medical Leave Act applies to all employees.
2. The Age Discrimination in Employment Act prohibits employment discrimination against individuals 50 years of age and older.
3. A prospective employer is restricted in the type of questions that can and cannot be asked during an interview.
4. Title VII of the Civil Rights Act only applies to race or color.
5. The Equal Pay Act guarantees that all employees will receive equal compensation.

Discussion Questions

1. Explain the progressive discipline model and when it might be used.
2. What are examples of standards of professionalism in health care? Which do you think are the most important?
3. If your personal values vary from those of a fellow employee, what problems might arise?
4. In your future healthcare career, with which type of professionals do you think you will have the most interaction?
5. Look up your professional code of ethics and list at least five standards that are specific to your profession.

REFERENCES

Hall v. Nalco Company, 534 F3d 644 (2008).

National Archives. (n.d.). *Teaching with documents: The Civil Rights Act of 1964 and the Equal Employment Opportunity Commission*. Retrieved from http://www.archives.gov/education/lessons/civil-rights-act/

Professional Association of Health Care Office Management. (2012). *Code of Ethics*. Retrieved from http://www.pahcom.com/membership/ethical_standards.html

United States Department of Health and Human Services. (2006). *Fact sheet*. Retrieved from http://www.hhs.gov/ocr/civilrights/resources/factsheets/504.pdf

United States Department of Labor. (2011). *Occupational Safety and Health Administration*. Retrieved from http://www.osha.gov/pls/oshaweb/owadisp.show_document?p_table=NEWS_RELEASES&p_id=19188

United States Department of Labor. (n.d.). *Healthcare facilities.* Retrieved from http://www.osha.gov/SLTC/healthcarefacilities/index.html

United States Department of Labor. (n.d.). *Health plans and benefits.* Retrieved from http://www.dol.gov/dol/topic/health-plans/cobra.htm

United States Department of Labor. (2010). *Wage and hour division.* Retrieved from http://www.dol.gov/whd/regs/compliance/hrg.htm

United States Equal Employment Opportunity Commission. (1997). *Filing a charge.* Retrieved from http://www.eeoc.gov/facts/howtofil.html

United States Equal Employment Opportunity Commission. (n.d.). *The Equal Pay Act of 1963.* Retrieved from http://www.eeoc.gov/laws/statutes/epa.cfm

Chapter 6

Accountability: The Medical Record

The pressure of adversity is the most powerful sustainer of accountability.

—Criss Jami
(poet, philosopher, and musician)
(Goodreads, n.d.)

In this chapter, you will learn about:

- The definition and purpose of a medical record
- The characteristics of proper documentation (FLOAT)
- The information that should be contained in the medical record
- Medical record ownership
- The Privacy Act of 1974
- Advantages of medical record information
- Advantages and disadvantages of a national electronic medical records system
- Two types of medical charting methods

Key terms

Electronic medical record (EMR)
Fidelity
FLOAT
Hopper

The Joint Commission (TJC)
Medical record
Narrative charting method
SOAP charting method
Subpoena duces tecum

For Your Consideration

Imagine the quality level of patient care without the medical record! It would be like starting over again each time the patient needs care. Think of all the potential mistakes in diagnoses, allergic reactions, and treatment plans (just to name a few). In short, health care without the medical record would turn the organization of the entire industry into utter chaos, no doubt resulting in the loss of many lives.

Think of your own medical history. What pieces of information contained within your record are essential in ongoing care and your best interests? Do not confine this information to medical conditions; consider age, family medical history, and even religious beliefs. Can you think of other details?

THE MEDICAL RECORD

The **medical record** is a written story of a patient's medical history **(Figure 6-1)**. It enables the physician to do the following:

- Assess family medical history
- Compare progress or lost ground in treatment
- Prescribe appropriate treatment plans
- Offer appropriate advice
- Refer to specialists
- Manage hospitalization, if necessary
- Manage information that could be used in the legal system

The medical record makes it possible for the healthcare professional to provide the most appropriate patient services. For example, the patient with more than one physician should be sure that all physicians involved in his or her care have the most current information so they can work together for the greatest benefit. A patient who switches from doctor to doctor is known as a **hopper**. Sometimes, patients go from doctor to doctor because they cannot find the satisfaction they are looking for in a healthcare provider. Sometimes, it may be because they owe money. Still other times, it is because they are seeking prescribed medications (e.g., pain medication). Advocates of a nationally standardized electronic medical records system contend that electronic records would virtually do away with a hopper.

The medical record is considered a legal document because the information in the record is often used as a primary source of evidence in lawsuits. Remember this in your everyday documentation practices because what you provide in writing could win or lose a legal case. If you are ever subpoenaed to be part of a case, you may have to defend what and how you have recorded information in a medical record. You

History	Performed	
	1 Introduces self.	
	2 Explains role of provider.	
	3 Opening question: What brings you in today?	I've got a cold.
Chronology/	4 When did it start?	About 3 days ago.
Onset	5 Was the onset sudden or gradual?	I guess gradual.
	6 Did you ever have this before?	I had the same thing last year.
Description	7 Describe the "cold."	I have a clear runny nose and sore throat.
Exacerbations	8 Anything make it worse?	It hurts more when I swallow.
Remittance	9 Anything make it better?	Some cold tablets I took helped.
Symptoms associated	10 Do you have any shortness of breath?	I just can't breathe through my nose.
	11 Fever or chills?	Both.
	12 Headache or sinus congestion/pressure?	Yes, right above my eyes.
	13 Do you have any visual changes?	No.
	14 Any ear pain?	No, they just feel full.
	15 Do you have a cough?	No.
Medical Hx	16 Do you have any other medical conditions?	No, I'm pretty healthy.
Medications	17 What medications are you on?	None.
Allergies	18 Do you have any allergies?	I'm allergic to amoxicillin.
	19 What happens when you take that?	I vomit.
Social Hx	20 Do you smoke?	No.
Menstrual Hx	21 When was the FDLNMP?	It started yesterday.
Surg/Hosp Hx	22 Have you had any surgeries or hospitalizations?	No.
Physical Exam	23 Informs patient that the physical exam is to begin.	
	24 Washes hands for 15 seconds.	
Vitals	25 Appropriately performed—if repeated measurements needed.	
General	26 General assessment	Alert, no respiratory distress.
Skin	27 Rash	None.
Head/Sinuses	28 Inspection, palpation	Normocephalic, atraumatic. Sinuses nontender
Eyes	29 Inspection	Conjunctive pink, sclera w/o injection

Figure 6-1 A medical record.

Source: Kauffman, M. (2007) *The History and Physical Examination Workbook: A Common Sense Approach*. Jones & Bartlett Learning, Burlington, MA, p. 141.

History	Performed	
Nose	30 Inspection	Mucosal edema and clear exudate
Ears	31 Inspection	TMs gray bilaterally, good light reflex
Mouth/Throat	32 Inspection	Pharyngeal erythema w/o exudate
Neck/Lymph	33 Inspection, palpation	Supple without masses, lymphadenopathy, or stiffness.
Lungs	34 Auscultation	Clear without wheezes, crackles
Cardiac	35 Auscultation: aortic, pulmonic, tricuspid, and mitral	Regular without murmur
Abdomen	36 Palpation	No splenomegaly.
Assessment/	37 Give three things in the differential diagnosis including URI.	
Plan	38 Explained likely etiology: Viral infection.	
	39 Explained plan: supportive therapy, throat culture, increase fluids, rest.	
	40 Asks the patient and family if they have any questions or suggestions.	
	41 Thanks the patient. Displayed professionalism and empathy.	

Figure 6-1 *Continued*

may later remember something that you did not include, but you will not be able to use that information once a subpoena has been issued.

Every institution or office may, to some degree, have its own practices about documentation, but every medical record should possess the following characteristics, which you can remember with the mnemonic **FLOAT**:

- Factual
- Legible
- Objective
- Accurate
- Timely

Factual

Since the medical record is a legal document, it is essential that it be factual. The information, if brought into a legal case, will be reviewed and possibly presented as evidence. The judge or jury will not be able to come to a conclusion on a point if it is not in the record. The phrase "not recorded . . . did not happen" will be enforced. Additionally, if you are about to perform a procedure (such as an injection), do not record until after you have completed the procedure.

Legible

How many times have people misinterpreted information because of poor handwriting? While it is widely known that many physicians do not have clear handwriting, it is often overlooked that many health-care professionals do not make extra efforts to write legibly. If people cannot read your writing, how can they assess patient information? If you find that your own handwriting is not the most legible, do what you can to improve it. Believe it or not, this could come up in a lawsuit.

Note that medical record entries should be done in blue or black ink only. Never make an entry in pencil or colored ink and never use erasable ink.

Physicians are now often choosing preprinted forms to save time and improve legibility issues. In such instances, physicians still must provide the time and date, and authenticate the information. As specified by the Centers for Medicare and Medicaid Services (2009), "Authentication of medical record entries may include written signatures, initials, computer key, or other code."

Case in Point: Dig a Little Deeper

Do an internet search on "physician sued for poor handwriting" and read some of the articles you find. You may be surprised to learn that many cases have been brought to suit as the result of poor handwriting.

Objective

The word objective suggests impartiality and fairness. It makes sense that the information contained in the medical record be objective. Personal opinions have no place in the medical record. For example, if the patient disagrees with a treatment plan offered, it would be unprofessional to record: "Patient was disagreeable to every option offered." Instead, proper documentation might include the following: "The patient was diagnosed with stage III liver cancer. Chemotherapy was refused. Radiation treatment was refused. Oncology referral was refused." The latter states what was offered and whether it was accepted. Terms such as "disagreeable" are subjective and do not belong in the record. Terms such as "every" or "never" are rarely true.

Consider the physician reviewing a new patient's medical record. If the record is clogged with personal comments and unnecessary information, it could hinder the assessments made in offering patient care. Always document as if you were trying to explain something very important to someone else: Be concise, but do not leave out any relevant details.

Accurate

The medical record is only as accurate as the efforts of those who record in it. The lack of accuracy, after all, can be the difference between a patient experiencing improved health and one experiencing a life-threatening situation. Spelling and grammar are also crucial. Accuracy does not refer just to the information either. Though it may seem obvious, you should always double-check to assure that you have the correct medical record before beginning to document—a simple, yet costly mistake.

Abbreviations are a controversial issue in charting. There are so many abbreviations that some could be confused. That is why professional organizations, educational institutions, and government agencies often have their own lists of approved abbreviations. The facility where you work should have an approved list on file and could even post some near work stations as reminders.

Words to the wise: Whether an unclear statement or a spelling mistake, a poorly written entry in the medical record can hinder accurate patient care **(Table 6-1)**.

Table 6-1 Record-Keeping Examples

Entry	Better Entry
Pt nonresponsive to questions	Pt did not give information on the following: last physical exam, last time he checked his own blood sugar levels, and amount of exercise.
Pt was given choice of prescriptions	Pt was given choice of sublingual B_{12} or a B_{12} injection. She chose the injection and was given 500 mcg.
Lover function seems normal	Liver function seems normal

Timely

Timeliness is of the essence in medical accountability. Let's face it, medical professionals usually have high patient loads, and it would be almost impossible to remember details of each patient without the aid of an accurate medical record. When you are with a patient, you should be making notes immediately to ensure the most accurate information. To do anything else is a disservice to the patient, and this reflects on your professionalism. According to the American Health Information Management Association, if you are not able to enter the information in a timely manner (meaning soon after the service was provided to the patient), you may add a late entry or an addendum, if it is clearly marked as such. Do not confuse a late entry or addendum, either of which is permitted, with information added unethically to enhance a medical record in preparation for court use. Unethical practices of adding information can result in punishment to the person making the entry (American Health Information Management Association, n.d.).

THE JOINT COMMISSION

The Joint Commission (TJC), a not-for-profit agency established in 1951, is an accreditation agency in the United States that reviews patient documentation. Its mission is "to continuously improve health care for the public, in collaboration with other stakeholders, by evaluating health care organizations and inspiring them to excel in providing safe and effective care of the highest quality and value" (TJC, 2012).

Despite what the name might suggest, the agency does not review only the records of hospitals. TJC also evaluates other patient service facilities such as dental offices, nursing homes, clinics, surgery facilities, and urgent care facilities. To earn and maintain TJC's "Gold Seal of Approval, an organization must undergo an on-site survey by a Joint Commission survey team at least every 3 years" (TJC, 2012). (Laboratories must be surveyed every 2 years.)

If a TJC representative visits your place of employment, remember that he or she is just there to help suggest improvements according to Gold Seal of Approval standards. Your best strategy is to cooperate fully. The representative will complete a written report of the audit, and your facility will be given time to make corrections. An audit can be a valuable learning experience so should your employer be audited, take the opportunity to learn from the experience and pay attention to the kinds of information that they are gathering, if you're able.

CONTENTS OF THE MEDICAL RECORD

Medical records, as stated earlier, provide a story of the patient's medical history, so consistency and content are of great significance. Though individual states vary regarding the specific information required, in general a satisfactory record will include the following:

- Each entry dated and initialed by person recording the information
- Insurance information (provider name and contact information)
- Patient's personal information (address, phone number, social security number, etc.)
- HIPAA forms
- X-rays, lab work, surgery records
- Medical history (including chief complaints and family medical history)
- Notes and charts recorded by the physician, physician assistant, nurse practitioner, or nurse

- Communications between healthcare providers
- Dates and times of appointments, and a record of missed appointments
- Telephone conversations between office staff or physician, dated
- Plans of actions/treatment plans (relating to diagnoses, hospitalization, referrals, treatments, therapy, prescriptions, etc.)

CORRECTING THE MEDICAL RECORD

Every person charting will, at some point, makes a writing mistake. When you make a mistake, you should never use correction fluid or erase the entry in any way. Instead, draw a thin line (also called a "strikethrough") through the mistake and write your initials and the date above the line. In doing so, the former statement can be seen in case there is any discrepancy.

TYPES OF MEDICAL RECORD CHARTING

There are several types of medical charting. Always follow the protocol of the facility where the patient's record is housed. We will discuss two common methods: the narrative method and the SOAP method.

The Narrative Method

The **narrative charting method** consists of thorough but concise documentation. At first glance, it may seem to be the easiest method, but in the long run, this method can make it quite difficult to decipher patient information and to fit all the information together to make decisions about patient care. Progress notes often are a part of this method.

The SOAP Method

The **SOAP charting method** often produces a more consistent record. SOAP is a mnemonic for the sections included in the record:

Subjective—The patient's chief complaints

Objective—The healthcare professional's observations and findings through examination and conversation

Assessment—Conclusions based on the subjective and objective information

Plan of action—The treatment that is advised based on the conclusions

By using this method, entries are easy to track throughout the record by category and, therefore, may even save time for the physician(s) reviewing it.

SENDING OUT MEDICAL INFORMATION

A patient's medical record should be carefully handled to protect the confidential nature of information contained in it. The preferred delivery method is through registered mail or through a reliable delivery service where a signature is required.

Faxing is a common way of sending medical information, but it should be used with great care. It, like e-mail, should be used only when the information is needed immediately and/or when other communication avenues are not feasible, and it should be used only with proper documentation of permission. Some states have laws that prohibit the faxing of medical information. Additionally, sending medical information by e-mail is quite risky, as unauthorized persons may be able to view it. The following are tips for faxing medical information (Myjer, 2003):

1. When the information is requested, verify that it is indeed going to a healthcare provider or is being sent as the result of a court order.
2. Make sure any information has a release of information signed by the physician approving that the information be sent and by the patient whose information is being shared.
3. When sending the fax, be sure the person requesting the information will be at the fax machine to receive the information. By doing so, you are preventing others from seeing the patient's medical record.
4. Only send the portion of the record that has been requested. If you send more, it could change the results of a court case. Only sending the portion requested is known as **subpoena duces tecum**, which is Latin for "bring with you under penalty of punishment."

5. Always be sure the fax number is correct before pushing the "send" button.

6. A cover sheet should always accompany the information, and it should be clearly and prominently marked "Confidential." Also, the following information should be included on the cover sheet:

   a. Date and time of transmission, along with number of pages (including cover page)

   b. Sender's name and name of facility, telephone number, and fax number

   c. Recipient information: name, facility, telephone number, fax number, and address

   d. A request for notification of receipt of information

   e. The patient's name, included on each page of the information except the cover page

---

Case Study: Frank Smith

Frank Smith works in a small factory. For the past couple of days, he has worked despite having a low-grade fever and abdominal pain, unbeknownst to his supervisor and coworkers. Finally, on the third day of his illness, he tells his supervisor, Linda Jonas, that he is ill and needs to go to the doctor. Frank was absent from work for a funeral just 2 weeks ago, and she does not really want him to leave but consents anyway.

Frank goes to his family physician, Dr. Price, who tells him that he has a virus that has been going around. The virus starts with a headache and then progresses to fever and abdominal pain. He is contagious and Dr. Price prescribes medication, advising bed rest for 2 more days. Frank has his wife take the doctor's excuse to his supervisor.

Ms. Jonas is upset that Frank is again absent from work and calls Dr. Price for details of Frank's condition. We learned in a previous case study that a physician may only discuss medical information with those listed in the patient's medical record. The question regarding this case study is, does the fact that Frank is contagious have any bearing on whether his information can be shared?

SHARING A PATIENT'S MEDICAL INFORMATION

Every patient has the right to have the details of his or her medical information protected, as specified by the Health Insurance Portability and Accountability Act (HIPAA). There are some exceptions, but for the most part, the patient decides who gets to see his or her personal medical information.

In the Frank Smith case study, he has the right to have details of his illness kept private. All the employer needs to know is that he has a doctor's excuse advising bed rest for 2 days. Even though Frank has a virus that is contagious, he does not have to disclose this to Ms. Jonas or anyone at his work unless he wishes to do so. If Frank had a case of whooping cough or another contagious condition listed by the Centers for Disease Control and Prevention (CDC) as sharable, Dr. Price would have had to share details of his condition with the local Health Department, who would then carry out usual procedures. However, the virus he has is not on the CDC's list, so no sharing of details is required. Frank should not lose his job for not sharing this information. Note that while Frank is not legally bound to report his virus to his employer, he may feel it ethically appropriate to report his contagious condition.

The purpose of confidentiality is to protect the patient. Reflecting upon this, you can rationalize that to further protect some patients, there are sometimes reasons why it is not good for the patient to have access to his or her own medical record. For example, the patient might do himself or herself harm, or the patient might be in an at-risk group (such as in the case of children, elderly patients who might not be capable of making sound decisions, or mental health patients).

Infectious Diseases Designated as Notifiable at the National Level During 2009 (CDC, 2009, 2011)[*]

Anthrax
Arboviral diseases, neuroinvasive and nonneuroinvasive
    California serogroup virus
    Eastern equine encephalitis virus

Powassan virus
St. Louis encephalitis virus
West Nile virus
Western equine encephalitis virus
Botulism
   Foodborne
   Infant
   Other (wound and unspecified)
Brucellosis
Chancroid
Chlamydia trachomatis infections
Cholera
Coccidioidomycosis
Cryptosporidiosis[†]
Cyclosporiasis
Diphtheria
Ehrlichiosis/Anaplasmosis
   Anaplasma phagocytophilum
   Ehrlichia chaffeensis
   Ehrlichia ewingii
   Undetermined
Giardiasis
Gonorrhea
Haemophilus influenzae, invasive disease
Hansen disease (Leprosy)
Hantavirus pulmonary syndrome
Hemolytic uremic syndrome, post-diarrheal
Hepatitis, viral, acute
Hepatitis, viral, chronic
Hepatitis A, acute
Hepatitis B, acute
Hepatitis B, chronic
Hepatitis B virus, perinatal infection
Hepatitis C, acute

Hepatitis C virus infection (past or present)
Human immunodeficiency virus (HIV) diagnosis[§]
Influenza-associated pediatric mortality
Legionellosis
Listeriosis
Lyme disease
Malaria
Measles[†]
Meningococcal disease
Mumps
Novel influenza A virus infections
Pertussis
Plague
Poliomyelitis, paralytic
Poliovirus infection, nonparalytic
Psittacosis
Q fever[†]
   Acute
   Chronic
Rabies
   Animal
   Human
Rocky Mountain spotted fever
Rubella[†]
Rubella, congenital syndrome
Salmonellosis
Severe acute respiratory syndrome-associated coronavirus
   (SARS-CoV) disease
Shiga toxin-producing *Escherichia coli* (STEC)
Shigellosis
Smallpox
Streptococcal disease, invasive, Group A
Streptococcal toxic-shock syndrome
Streptococcus pneumoniae, drug resistant, all ages, invasive disease

Streptococcus pneumoniae, invasive disease non-drug resistant,
    in children 5 years of age and younger
Syphilis
Syphilis, congenital
Tetanus
Toxic-shock syndrome (other than streptococcal)
Trichinellosis
Tuberculosis[†]
Tularemia
Typhoid fever
Vancomycin-intermediate *Staphylococcus aureus* (VISA) infection
Vancomycin-resistant *Staphylococcus aureus* (VRSA) infection
Varicella (morbidity)
Varicella (mortality)
Vibriosis
Yellow fever

---

[*] Position statements of the Council of State and Territorial Epidemiologists approved in 2008 for national surveillance were implemented beginning in January 2009. No new conditions were added to the notifiable disease list in 2009.

[†] In a 2009 position statement, the Council of State and Territorial Epidemiologists approved the modified national tuberculosis surveillance case definition.

[§] AIDS has been reclassified as HIV stage III.

ELECTRONIC MEDICAL RECORDS

No doubt, the issue of digitalizing medical records has been one of controversy. The **electronic medical record (EMR)** is a medical record documented on and available by computer. It is also referred to as an EHR (electronic health record).

Those against EMRs argue that the system would be vulnerable to hackers and that any altered records could jeopardize the health, and possibly the very life, of the patient. After all, critics of the EMR system maintain, if the computer systems of the U.S. Pentagon can be hacked into, then surely an EMR system could fall prey to intruders.

Those who support the EMR system argue that such a system would allow for more efficient collaboration between physicians and that the system would be quicker to access than having to request and then wait to receive written records. The issue of legibility discussed in this chapter would become a nonfactor, though spelling mistakes would remain a problem.

Whether you do or do not support an EMR system, one is on its way. The U.S. federal government has mandated that by the year 2015, each medical facility must provide evidence of "meaningful use" of an EMR system, as prescribed by the state of location. There are incentives by some states for those who comply early. There will also be penalties (such as a reduction in Medicare payment) to those who do not comply (MedicalRecords.com, n.d.).

Case Study: Angelica Diaz

Angelica Diaz is originally from Guatemala. She recently became a U.S. citizen but speaks very little English. The U.S. Department of Health and Human Services has just begun a National Electronic Health Record System (NEHRS). Angelica learned about the NEHRS from her sister, who came to America 10 years ago and speaks fluent English.

Angelica has been having a lot of pain in her pelvic area, so much so that she has not been able to work for over a week. Her sister finally convinces her to go to a family physician, Dr. Reynolds.

There is a problem: Angelica engaged in prostitution when she first came to this country and was arrested. Fearing further humiliation, she does not tell her doctor that she has gonorrhea. She is afraid that she will suffer prejudice if others know, believing that too many people may be able to view her EMR. Dr. Reynolds asks Angelica a series of questions, but she is vague in her answers.

What are the possible ethical implications in this case? What consequences could not being honest with the physician have on her health? What strategies could the NEHRS put in place to help prevent these kinds of problems for the benefit of the patient?

ETHICAL CONSIDERATIONS OF THE EMR

How secure is the EMR? What precautions are to be taken to ensure that only authorized persons view a medical record? Does the patient lose control of his or her own medical information if it is digitized? These and many other questions are often brought up when debating the use of a standardized EMR. Consider the following ethical principles as they relate to the EMR (Layman, 2008).

- *Autonomy.* Autonomy is a person's ability to make decisions concerning his or her own personal well-being, including health care. If the EMR is accessible to, say, all hospitals in the case of an emergency, does the patient still have the autonomy to decide who can view the EMR?
- *Trust.* If a patient fears that the EMR might fall into the wrong hands, that patient might be less likely to fully disclose health information. Examples of information that might be withheld include pain level and disability.
- *Justice.* Would all people have equal access to EMRs, including those of lower socioeconomic status and those who do not speak English? If the EMR is to be a government-sanctioned system, then should it not consider equity among all patients?
- *Fidelity.* **Fidelity** in the field of ethics simply means loyalty. Is fidelity to be questioned if the record is susceptible to documentation mistakes and thievery (hackers)?

If the patient feels compromised in regard to any of these ethical principles, might he or she hesitate in seeking medical treatment? What do you think?

American Medical Association Statement: E-7.05
Retention of Medical Records

Physicians have an obligation to retain patient records which may reasonably be of value to a patient. The following guidelines are offered to assist physicians in meeting their ethical and legal obligations: (1) Medical considerations are the primary basis for deciding how long to retain medical records. For example, operative notes and chemotherapy records should always be part of the patient's chart. In deciding whether to keep certain parts of the record, an appropriate criterion is whether a physician would want the information if he or she were seeing the patient for the first time. (2) If a particular record no longer needs to be kept for medical reasons, the physician should check state laws to see if there is a requirement that records be kept for a minimum length of time. Most states will not have such a provision. If they do, it will be part of the statutory code or state licensing board. (3) In all cases, medical records should be kept for at least as long as the length of time of the statute of limitations for medical malpractice claims. The statute of limitations may be three or more years, depending on the state law. State medical associations and insurance carriers are the best resources for this information. (4) Whatever the statute of limitations, a physician should measure time from the last professional contact with the patient. (5) If a patient is a minor, the statute of limitations for medical malpractice claims may not apply until the patient reaches the age of majority. (6) Immunization records always must be kept. (7) The records of any patient covered by Medicare or Medicaid must be kept at least five years. (8) In order to preserve confidentiality when discarding old records, all documents should be destroyed. (9) Before discarding old records, patients should be given an opportunity to claim the records or have them sent to another physician, if it is feasible to give them the opportunity. (IV, V) Issued June 1994. (American Medical Association, n.d.)

PUTTING IT ALL TOGETHER

The medical record contains vital information about the patient, aiding the healthcare team in providing the best patient care. The well-maintained medical record is characterized by the mnemonic FLOAT: factual, legible, objective, accurate, and timely. Never make changes that erase original entries. Instead, draw a line through the entry, make the correction, then date and initial the new entry. Use black or blue ink, never red or another color of ink, and never record with a pencil or erasable ink. Improperly altering a medical record is illegal because the medical record is considered a legal document.

The EMR is certainly in the future big picture of medical record keeping, though there are concerns that it could take away some degree of autonomy, justice, trust, and fidelity. However, advocates of an EMR system maintain that it would offer consistency and faster access to patient records for faster care, and would do away with the hopper (a person who switches from doctor to doctor).

Since the medical record is considered a legal document, it should be consistent and concise (but thorough). Remember that every entry is susceptible to being brought up as evidence in a court of law. Knowing this should help you appreciate the great weight held by the medical record.

The fewer people who handle a medical record, the greater the chance of protecting patient confidentiality. The most trusted method of sending a record is using registered mail or using a reliable delivery service and requiring a delivery signature. When you do have to send something immediately, you may be called upon to fax documents. When doing so, remember these guidelines:

- Only send the portion requested
- Be sure to verify that the requester is a healthcare provider or is requesting the information as the result of a legal action
- Confirm that the requester will be at the receiving fax machine to ensure that the information is safe in the correct hands
- Include a cover letter
- Check the fax number for accuracy
- Be sure the release of information documents have been signed and are filed in the patient's medical record.

The medical record should be protected because it can contain the most personal and fragile of data about a person. Never leave a record where others can read it, and always file it away as soon as possible. Your diligence in appropriate charting can ensure exemplary patient care and documentation that will clearly tell a story if needed in any legal action.

CHAPTER CHECKUP

Fill-in-the-Blanks

1. _____, put simply, means loyalty.
2. A _____ is a person who switches from doctor to doctor.
3. TJC stands for _____ _____ _____.
4. The medical record is considered a legal _____.

Listing

1. There are seven advantages offered through the medical record. List them:
2. The SOAP method of medical charting is commonly used. List what SOAP stands for and explain.
3. List four ethical issues concerning the electronic medical record (EMR):
4. The FLOAT method reminds the healthcare professional of five preferable characteristics of a medical record. List and explain each.

REFERENCES

American Health Information Management Association. (n.d.). *Legal document standards*. Retrieved from http://www.ahima.org/resources/infocenter/ltc/guide5.aspx

American Medical Association. (n.d.). E-7.05 Retention of medical records. Retrieved from https://ssl3.ama-assn.org/apps/ecomm/PolicyFinderForm.pl?site=www.ama-assn.org&uri=%2fresources%2fdoc%2fPolicyFinder%2fpolicyfiles%2fHnE%2fE-7.05.HTM

Centers for Disease Control and Prevention. (2009). *Morbidity and Mortality Weekly Report*: Summary of notifiable diseases—United States (2009). Retrieved from http://www.cdc.gov/mmwr/PDF/wk/mm5853.pdf

Centers for Disease Control and Prevention. (2011, May 13). Summary of notifiable diseases—United States, 2009. *Morbidity and Mortality Weekly Report, 58*(53), 3.

Centers for Medicare and Medicaid Services, Department of Health and Human Services. (2009). *Appendix A, Interpretive guidelines for hospitals* (revised). (Publication No. 100-07). Retrieved from http://health .nv.gov/HCQC/R47SOMA.pdf

Goodreads *Quotes about accountability*. (n.d.). Retrieved from http://www .goodreads.com/quotes/tag/accountability

Layman, E. J. (2008). Ethical issues and the electronic health record. National Institutes of Health: US National Library of Medicine. *PubMed, 27*(2), 165–176. Retrieved from http://www.ncbi.nlm.nih.gov/ pubmed/18475119

MedicalRecords.com. (n.d.). Electronic medical records deadline: Will I be assessed penalties for not using an EMR system? Retrieved from http://www.medicalrecords.com/physicians/electronic-medical-records-deadline

Myjer, D. (2003). Policy on fax, e-mail protects privacy. *Stanford Hospital and clinics update: Medical staff update*. Retrieved from http://med.stanford .edu/shs/update/archives/JUNE2003/privacy.html

The Joint Commission. (2012). About the Joint Commission. Retrieved from http://www.jointcommission.org/about_us/history.aspx

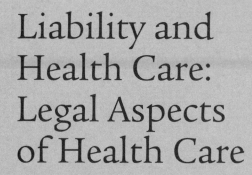

Chapter 7

Liability and Health Care: Legal Aspects of Health Care

*Laws are not invented.
They grow out of
circumstances.*

—Azarias

IN THIS CHAPTER, YOU WILL LEARN ABOUT:

- Various sources of law in the United States and how they affect healthcare professionals
- The difference between intentional and unintentional torts
- The PYTHON principle
- Liability and the impact it has on healthcare professionals

KEY TERMS

Administrative law	Duty
Assault and battery	Embezzlement
Assumption of risk	False imprisonment
Borrowed servant rule	Fraud
Breach of duty	Invasion of privacy
Causation	Liability insurance
Civil action	Malfeasance
Common law	Misfeasance
Constitutional law	Negligence
Contributory and	Nonfeasance
comparative negligence	PYTHON principle
Criminal action	Scope of practice
Damages	Statute of limitations
Denial	Statutory law
Defamation of character	Tort (intentional and
Doctrine of *res ipsa loquitur*	unintentional)
Doctrine of *respondeat superior*	

For Your Consideration

Most employees follow rules because they want to keep their jobs and avoid punishments. As healthcare professionals, we also have an ethical obligation to protect our patients from potential harm. Having a knowledge and understanding of the laws that surround health care is essential to protect both yourself and your patients.

SOURCES OF LAW

To properly understand legal aspects of health care, it is important to recognize the various sources of laws. In the United States, laws originate from three primary sources: the Constitution, the judicial system, and the federal and state governments. These sources are interrelated and are not easily separated, so it is necessary to have an understanding of the origins of each.

Constitutional Law

The U.S. Constitution is considered the highest law in our country. It outlines the rights and responsibilities of the federal government, state governments, and individuals. Any new law written must comply with the Constitution. If a law is found to be unconstitutional, it cannot be upheld. A current issue that has been challenged is that of the forced purchase of health insurance. In August of 2011, the 11th Circuit Court of Appeals in Atlanta, Georgia, ruled that the government is not allowed to force U.S. citizens to purchase healthcare insurance (Kane, 2011). This mandate was part of the 2010 Affordable Care Act signed into law by President Obama. The basis for this judgment is that forcing citizens to purchase insurance oversteps the bounds of the Constitution's Commerce Clause. The Commerce Clause allows the government to create certain programs that regulate economic activity. The Supreme Court was called upon to decide on this case.

Common Law

Under the guidelines of the Constitution, our federal government has three branches: executive (presidential), legislative (senate and representatives), and judicial (courts) **(Figure 7-1)**. States also have their own governmental systems, which include a judicial branch. **Common law** is set by the judicial branch. The outcome of court cases establishes common law. For example, in the landmark case of Roe vs. Wade, the federal Supreme Court established the common law right to privacy regarding reproductive rights for women. At the state level, the Oregon Supreme Court upheld the common law right to privacy regarding a patient's right to choose his or her method of death.

Administrative Law

The federal government can create agencies and give them the right to implement certain laws. These laws are known as regulatory or **administrative law**. Some agencies that implement laws related to

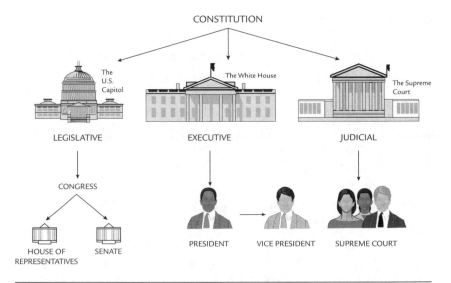

Figure 7-1 Branches of government and sources of law.
Source: Superintendent of Documents, U.S. Government Printing Office.

health care include the Food and Drug Administration, the Office of Civil Rights (oversees violations to the Health Insurance Portability and Accountability Act [HIPAA]), and the Department of Health and Human Services. A specific administrative law that pertains to healthcare providers is the Controlled Substances Act. This law is part of the Comprehensive Drug Abuse Prevention and Control Act of 1970 and gives authority to the Drug Enforcement Agency and the Department of Health and Human Services to categorize drugs into schedules that determine who is authorized to administer and obtain those drugs. These rules have the effect of law.

Statutory Law

The federal and state governments also create their own laws. These laws start as bills, must be approved by both legislative branches (Senate and House of Representatives), and must eventually be signed by the president (federal laws) or governor (state laws). The president and governors also have the right to issue executive orders. All **statutory laws** and executive orders must comply with the Constitution. An example of a statutory law is the Good Samaritan laws. These laws are specific to states and generally provide immunity to ordinary citizens who assist victims in an emergency. Some states, such as Minnesota, use wording that suggests citizens have a duty to assist, while other states only provide immunity if they choose to assist. Another example of a statutory law would be those created by states that require healthcare professionals to report suspected cases of abuse. These are generally known as mandatory reporting laws.

Statutory law can be divided into two main categories: civil and criminal. A **criminal action** is considered a wrong against society. A **civil action** is considered a wrong between individuals. It is important to note that an action can be both criminal and civil. Criminal cases can result in confinement, probation, or community service. Civil cases can result in fines, usually paid to the victim or victim's family, or the order to perform a specific action, such as keeping pets under control. If a case is tried as both a criminal and a civil case, the criminal trial is generally held first, followed by the civil. Criminal cases require the trier of fact, usually a jury, to find the defendant guilty "beyond a reasonable doubt," while civil cases require only a preponderance of evidence.

Case in Point: Good Samaritan Home

In Albert Lea, Minnesota, several nursing aides were charged with various criminal actions including disorderly conduct by a healthcare provider. The nursing aides (all teenagers at the time) reportedly verbally and physically abused elderly patients at the Good Samaritan Home. In addition to the criminal charges, the families of the victims alleged negligence by the Good Samaritan Home, claiming the nursing aides were not properly supervised. The criminal trial resulted in a guilty verdict for all the defendants with various sentences, including jail time. The civil suit was settled out of court.

Some statutory laws provide remedies for wrongs committed against society or individuals. Wrongs against individuals are called **torts**. Torts can be divided into two main categories: intentional and unintentional. **Intentional torts** that are most common in health care include assault and battery, false imprisonment, defamation of character, invasion of privacy, fraud, and embezzlement.

- **Assault and battery**: Historically, assault meant the threat of harm, and battery was the actual physical harm to a person. Currently, most states consider both the threat and the act to come under the single term of assault. This includes unwanted touching. In the preceding Good Samaritan Home example, the teenage perpetrators were likely liable in the civil suit for committing intentional torts against the victims due to unwanted touching. While violent physical acts upon a person do occasionally happen in healthcare settings, most assault cases involve unwanted touching or performing a procedure without consent. Patients generally sign consent forms before having any medical procedure. Oral consent is also considered legally binding but can be much more difficult to prove in court. If a patient agrees to a procedure, he or she must be told if there will be any changes to that procedure prior to the change (e.g., additional tissue removed, change of surgeon). Changing procedures or medical professionals without consent damages the healthcare provider–patient relationship and can result in lack of trust. If the patient is not informed of these changes and the procedures are completed, the provider can be charged with assault.

- **False imprisonment**: Holding a patient against his or her will is considered false imprisonment. This includes the use of restraints for nonmedically approved reasons.
- **Defamation of character**: Defamation of character occurs when a person's reputation is damaged by the spreading of untrue information. While gossiping about coworkers or patients is unethical, if the information is true, it is not defamation of character. Defamation of character has two subcategories: slander and libel. Slander is spoken, and libel is written.
- **Invasion of privacy**: The intrusion into the private life of another person without medical cause can be considered invasion of privacy. This is different than a violation of HIPAA's Privacy Rule because invasion of privacy extends farther than protected health information. Any damaging information that is made public regarding any employee or patient in a healthcare setting can be considered invasion of privacy.
- **Fraud**: Deceitful practices that deprive someone of his or her rights can be considered fraud. Fraud can occur in many ways in health care. False promises, upcoding, and insurance fraud are only a few examples. Upcoding involves charging insurance companies for a procedure that is reimbursed at a higher rate than the procedure that was actually performed. An example of upcoding would be if a therapist meets with several patients in a group but bills the sessions individually, rather than as a group therapy session. Individual therapy sessions are generally reimbursed at a higher rate than group

therapy sessions. Medicaid and Medicare fraud has also become quite common and costly to taxpayers. In particular, you should never promise an outcome to a patient because, as we all know, no outcome is ever guaranteed. For example, you have a patient, Mrs. Lee, who has been a patient at the clinic where you work for more than 20 years and has always been kind and likeable, even when she is ill. She has just been told that she has cancer, and you are sad about this. You go into the examination room with Mrs. Lee and she reaches out for a hug. As you hug her, you say, "Don't worry, Mrs. Lee. We are going to beat this cancer." If you make a statement like this or any statement that promises a particular outcome, you have risked a possible lawsuit. Promises not kept in health care are considered fraud and can be brought to legal action as an intentional tort, even if you mean well. *Always be careful of your words and actions; they can come back to haunt you if you have acted improperly.*

- **Embezzlement**: The conversion to your own use of property that you can rightly access but do not own can be considered embezzlement. Generally, this involves an employee taking money from business accounts to which the employee has rightful access. Embezzlement is not the same as stealing because in cases of embezzlement, the employee has legal access to the funds, but chooses to take some for his or her personal use.

Case in Point: Mohr vs. Williams

In the landmark case of Mohr vs. Williams, the plaintiff (Mohr) was scheduled to have the defendant (Williams, an ear specialist) operate on her right ear. During the surgery, Williams decided that Mohr's left ear, rather than the right ear, required surgery. This condition was not life threatening and the surgery on the left ear was successful. Because Williams did not obtain consent from Mohr to operate on the left ear, Mohr brought a case of battery against Williams. The trial court found in favor of Mohr due to lack of consent. Performing a procedure without consent is considered battery. In emergency situations, doctors can rely on implied consent (an understanding that if the patient could give consent, he or she would do so), but in nonemergency situations, consent must be obtained before performing any medical procedure. (*Mohr v. Williams*, 1905)

Unintentional torts are commonly known as negligence. **Negligence** can occur in any field where a duty is owed to someone. Once healthcare professionals are licensed, they become legally liable for their employment actions. All healthcare professionals must uphold an appropriate standard of care. Standard of care is determined by what other professionals would reasonably do in a similar situation. There are four components necessary for an unintentional tort to bring a successful claim: duty, breach of duty, causation, and damages.

- **Duty** is established when a healthcare professional agrees to treat a patient. The standard of care for healthcare professionals is determined by what other members of the same profession would do in a similar situation.
- **Breach of duty** is the failure of a healthcare professional to act as any ordinary and prudent healthcare professional within the same community would act in similar circumstances. If the outcome of a procedure is one that the patient did not anticipate or was not informed about, then this may constitute negligence. Breaches fall under three general categories: **Misfeasance** occurs when a mistake is made (e.g., giving the patient the wrong medication). **Nonfeasance** is a failure to act (e.g., forgetting to turn a patient, which results in bed sores). **Malfeasance** is negligence with mal-intent (e.g., holding a noncooperative patient too tightly when drawing blood, which results in bruising).

- **Causation** requires the injury to be closely related to the healthcare professional's negligence. The patient is required to prove that the healthcare professional's breach was the direct cause of the injury that resulted. Put simply, the patient must prove that there were no other circumstances that could have caused the same injury. For instance, if a patient loses feeling in her arm after a blood sample was taken, she must prove that there was no other cause—such as a car accident or sports injury—that occurred between the time the blood was drawn and the time the nerve damage happened. This is one reason that keeping careful medical records is important. If a patient claims to have been seen by a medical assistant on a certain day at a certain time, the medical assistant should be able to confirm or dispute that claim.
- **Damages** are the actual injuries caused by the defendant for which compensation is due.

Many unintentional torts are brought against not only the employee charged with the negligent act, but also the employer. This is due to the **doctrine of *respondeat superior*** ("let the master answer"), which states that employers are responsible for employees' actions **(Figure 7-2)**. This responsibility includes training of employees, oversight of medical care, and financial compensation to injured parties, as appropriate. In the preceding Good Samaritan Home example, the hospital would likely be liable for negligence in failing to supervise the teens working as aides in the facility. If a plaintiff chooses to make a claim against the employer and is successful, the employer can seek to recover the damages from the employee who committed the negligent act.

In most cases, the plaintiff carries the burden of proof in claiming to be a victim of an unintentional tort. If the negligent act is so obvious that it appears there could be no other responsible party, the burden of proof shifts to the defendant, who must prove that he or she is not responsible for the injury. These cases are brought under the **doctrine of *res ipsa loquitur*** ("the thing speaks for itself"). Some common examples include amputation of the wrong limb or sponges

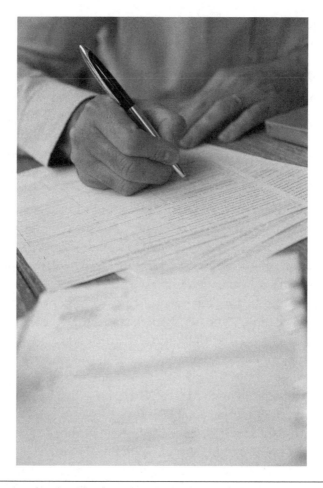

Figure 7-2 Under the doctrine of *respondeat superior*, the physician assumes responsibility of each of his or her employees and is therefore liable for any wrongdoings.

left in the body after surgery; it is obvious that the healthcare worker or workers were at fault, as no one else could have caused the injury.

If a healthcare professional is blamed in a tort, there are certain defenses he or she can raise, including denial, assumption of risk, comparative and contributory negligence, statute of limitations, and borrowed servant.

- **Denial** is the most commonly used defense in cases of negligence. The defendant does not claim that damages did not occur, but rather that there was another explanation or cause for the damages.
- **Assumption of risk** is the understanding that certain procedures can result in commonly known injuries. When patients give permission for certain procedures or refuse the medical advice of healthcare professionals, they are usually asked to sign consent forms to show that they understand the risks involved.
- In **contributory negligence** the patient or others are determined to be fully or in part responsible for the injury. In this case, they are not able to receive monetary compensation for damages. An example is if a patient falls when attempting to get out of bed independently after the patient was told not to get out of bed independently. Similar to contributory negligence, **comparative negligence** states that the plaintiff's actions helped cause the injury. The difference is that the plaintiff can recover damages based on the amount of the defendant's fault. So, if $100,000 was determined to be the monetary damages and the physician was 60% at fault, the patient could receive $60,000.
- **Statutes of limitations** determine the number of years a plaintiff has to file a claim of negligence. In medical malpractice cases, the statute of limitations begins at the time the injury is discovered. States have their own statutes of limitations, but in general they are 3 to 7 years.
- The **borrowed servant rule** is generally used by employers that have temporary workers or medical professionals who fill in for other medical professionals on leave. If a plaintiff sues a healthcare facility regarding the actions of an employee on temporary employment, the facility might utilize the borrowed servant rule and escape liability for injury caused by the temporary employee.

LIABILITY INSURANCE

Liability insurance provides financial protection from claims that arise from patients who believe they have been a victim of medical malpractice while under the care of a healthcare professional (Mello, 2006). Most healthcare providers need to buy some form of professional liability insurance. States generally require that physicians have liability insurance or work for a medical group that shares a liability plan. Physicians will generally carry liability insurance that includes a rider that covers the employees under them. Other healthcare professionals should check with their employer to see if they are covered by a general liability policy or if they are responsible for obtaining their own **(Figure 7-3)**. Some professional organizations, such as the American Association of Medical Assistants and the American Speech-Language and Hearing Association, offer liability insurance at a group rate for members. It is important to note that healthcare professionals need to protect their assets as well as

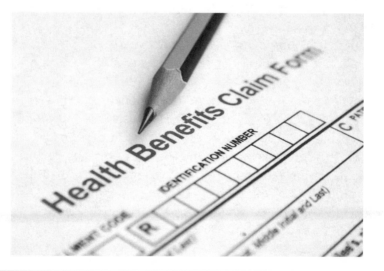

Figure 7-3 Healthcare professionals should consider carrying liability insurance or make sure they are covered by their employer's policy.

professional standing by obtaining some type of liability insurance. No matter how well a healthcare professional upholds the appropriate standard of care, mistakes can happen. Also, healthcare professionals can be accused in a lawsuit even when they are not guilty of any wrongdoing.

Case in Point: Hall vs. Hilbun

In the landmark case of Hall vs. Hilbun, Dr. Hilbun (defendant) surgically removed an abdominal obstruction from Terry Hall (plaintiff). After surgery, Hilbun accompanied Hall back to her room and left her in the care of the nurses on duty. During the night, Hall complained to the nurses of abdominal pain, but they did not contact Hilbun. Hilbun did not follow up on Hall's condition. In the early morning, Hall's condition deteriorated and Hilbun was contacted. By the time he reached the hospital, Hall had died. An autopsy showed that a sponge was left in Hall's abdominal cavity after the surgery, but it did not contribute to her death.

The four components of negligence are present in this case. Hilbun had a duty to provide an appropriate standard of care to Terry Hall, including follow-up instructions and visits. Hilbun breached this duty when he did not follow up on Hall's condition or ask nurses to call him if Hall had certain symptoms. This lack of care, not the sponge itself, is likely the direct cause of her death. In addition to her death, other damages include possible lack of income and companionship to her survivors. Under the doctrine of *respondeat superior*, Hilbun is held to a higher standard of liability because he is responsible for the actions of the nurses. (*Hall v. Hilbun*, 1985)

SCOPE OF PRACTICE

In your upcoming healthcare career, you will be charged with possessing specific skills and knowledge to properly do your job. The boundaries of what you can and cannot do and the regulations (as determined by your profession, your state, and the federal government) that dictate these boundaries are called your **scope of practice**. Therefore, let us define scope of practice as limitations, rules, and professional protocol that control what is proper within a given field.

Let's consider, for example, the medical office receptionist (MOR). The MOR's job responsibilities could include the following:

- Receiving patients
- Making sure patients sign in and that their information is promptly removed from the sign-in area for confidentiality purposes
- If the patient is new, distributing patient information forms, including the HIPAA forms, and having the patient complete and return them
- Making patient appointments

The MOR should only be performing duties specific to that job. Further, the MOR should not be performing duties that are suited to, say, the medical assistant. Logically, the MOR would not be trained or skilled at conducting physician duties such as giving diagnoses or referring a patient to a specialist. There may be times when a coworker needs the MOR's assistance, and this is perfectly acceptable as long as he or she has been trained to perform any duties before doing them. The entire healthcare team in a clinic, hospital, or any medical facility should work together to deliver the highest level of professionalism possible.

For Your Consideration

---

1. Think about your upcoming healthcare career and list the responsibilities of your intended profession.
2. Now list the responsibilities of another healthcare profession that might be closely related to yours. Hint: You may need to do an internet search to find job responsibilities in making these lists.
3. Compare the similarities and the differences between the lists.
4. Imagine each list in a box of its own. The responsibilities in that box could be regarded as the scope of practice for that particular profession. Think about it: You will be trained and gain practice in the responsibilities in *your* box—not other boxes. Therefore, it is reasonable that you should only perform the skills listed in your scope of practice box. Performing skills from another box could result in mistakes and, worse yet, a hurt patient. Of major concern also, you could be involved in legal action.
5. By remembering this "box exercise," you should more easily remember the importance of staying within your scope of practice.

THE PYTHON PRINCIPLE

The wise healthcare professional knows that preventing a lawsuit is a constant effort. Every time you come into contact with a patient, there is a chance of oversight that could trigger legal action. Commencement of legal action does not always end in liability or a guilty verdict, but it is better to avoid the chance. The **PYTHON principle** is an easy way to posture yourself for prevention. It was developed by one of the authors of this text, Carla Stanford, to

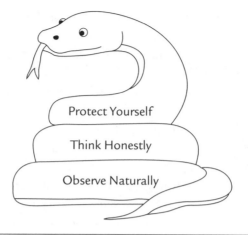

Figure 7-4 The PYTHON principle: safeguarding yourself from legal action.
Source: Developed by Carla C. Stanford, PhD (2009).

remind college students in healthcare majors how to prevent risk of legal action. It stands for Protect Yourself; Think Honestly; Observe Naturally **(Figure 7-4)**.

Protecting yourself means you are aware of the various ways you could be held liable as a legal professional. For example, if you send a fax containing confidential information to anyone, you put yourself at risk of breaching confidentiality. To prevent this, be sure a consent form has been signed and dated by the patient.

Honesty is a building block in the foundation of ethics. Honest dealings with patients, coworkers, employers, and even the legal system will help prevent future complications. Imagine a physical therapy assistant overhearing a physical therapist promising a stroke victim that therapy will "have them up on their feet in no time." This could be considered fraud. If the physical therapist is called to testify during the trial, she might be tempted by loyalty to the coworker to lie or omit the statement, but the physical therapy assistant has an ethical and legal obligation to cooperate with the legal system and tell the truth. If the assistant is not truthful, she puts herself at risk for loss of license, as well as her job. Honesty is always the best ethical and legal choice. The healthcare professional should never promise results. In caring for human beings, many factors come into play, making any outcome unpredictable.

Observations are critical for all healthcare professionals. Keeping track of observations and taking them all into consideration can help prevent legal action. For instance, if a nursing assistant observes that a patient is frequently coughing during meals, he or she can report this to the speech therapist on staff. An evaluation might determine that the patient has a choking risk and should have diet changes recommended. Being proactive can prevent legal action against the healthcare facility. It is always better to make an effort to prevent any wrongdoing than to try to defend it in the court of law.

PUTTING IT ALL TOGETHER

Since we are just covering the basics of the U.S. justice system, you should familiarize yourself with the three branches of government as well as the four types of laws. Understanding that the healthcare professional can be the target of a lawsuit should remind you to be at your professional best every day and to remember that the welfare of the patient is the foremost job of the healthcare professional.

In your career, you may never become involved in a lawsuit, but it is likely that someone you know in your field will. It is imperative that you know the laws, both federal and state, and that you keep up with the basics of those laws. You can keep up with many current events through the national and state professional organizations within your field, such as the American Association of Medical Assistants.

If you focus on your duties within your scope of practice, you will be less likely to be at risk for legal action, but keep in mind that anyone can be sued. Being sued does not automatically establish guilt. That is why it is important to be alert and document patient information well—not only what you did do (e.g., injections, medications) but what you did not do (e.g., patient's missed appointments, patient's refusal for treatment).

CHAPTER CHECKUP

Listing

1. List the four sources of law in the U.S. justice system.
2. Breaches fall under three general categories. List the three and define them.

Fill-in-the-Blanks

1. _____ actions are crimes against society, while _____ actions are crimes against one or more individuals.
2. Assault and battery, false imprisonment, and embezzlement are examples of _____ _____.
3. Damage that is caused to a person's reputation through spoken or written word by spreading untrue information is called _____ or _____.
4. *Respondeat superior* means _____ the _____ _____.

Discussion

1. Discuss the differences between unintentional and intentional torts.
2. Explain the borrowed servant rule.
3. Explain what the PYTHON principle is and what it means to healthcare professionals.

REFERENCES

Hall v. Hilbun, Supreme Court of Mississippi, 466 So.2d 856 (1985).

Kane, J. (2011, August 12). Americans can't be forced to buy insurance, 11th Circuit rules. *The Rundown*. Retrieved from http://www.pbs.org/news-hour/rundown/2011/08/americans-cant-be-forced-to-buy-insurance-11th-circuit-rules.html

Mello, M. (2006). Understanding medical malpractice insurance: A primer. Retrieved from http://www.rwjf.org/pr/synthesis/reports_and_briefs/pdf/no8_primer.pdf

Mohr v. Williams, Minnesota Supreme Court, 104 N.W. 12 (1905).

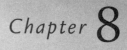

Chapter 8

Life and Death Issues

Ethics is nothing less than reverence for life.

—Albert Schweitzer

Dying is a part of living—a natural progression. Should I ignore the natural order of my life, twist it to my liking and thereby become something I was not meant to be?

—Charles de Lint
(*The Little Country*)

IN THIS CHAPTER, YOU WILL LEARN ABOUT:

- Issues surrounding end-of-life care
- The importance of advance directives
- Legal and ethical options for patients and families making decisions about end-of-life care
- Issues surrounding fertility options
- Legal and ethical issues surrounding the beginning of life

KEY TERMS

Abortion	Hospice
Active euthanasia	In vitro fertilization
Artificial insemination	Living will
Assisted reproduction	Medical power of attorney
Beneficence	Palliative care
Conscience clause	Passive euthanasia
Curative care	Persistent vegetative state
Euthanasia	Surrogacy
Healthcare proxy	Uniform Anatomical Gift Act

For Your Consideration

Not all healthcare professionals will deal with patients facing life-or-death issues. At some point, however, we will all encounter someone who is facing an issue related to the beginning or the end of life. In an effort to be a well-rounded healthcare professional, it is important to understand all sides of these issues. With understanding comes the ability to provide compassionate care.

ETHICAL ISSUES RELATED TO DYING

An 87-year-old widow, Evelyn, checked into the emergency department complaining of abdominal pain. Shortly after admission, it became clear that Evelyn was confused and unable to make decisions for herself. During the past 3 years, she has had two surgeries related to diverticulitis and abdominal cancer. Evelyn also suffers from severe back and leg pain, which has recently been diagnosed as sciatic nerve pain. After consulting her medical record, the attending physician determines that Evelyn has two advance directives on file. The directives are a living will and a designation of her only son as a healthcare proxy. It is decided that Evelyn and her son should meet with the hospital's ethics committee to discuss options.

While not all healthcare professionals will interact with patients who have life-and-death decisions to make, we all know or have known someone who is dying. It is important for all healthcare professionals and consumers to know the rights and ethical issues surrounding death. When it is determined that a patient, like Evelyn, has certain medical conditions, such as diverticulitis and cancer, the first intervention is generally curative care. **Curative care** is any care given in an effort to cure or reduce a medical problem. At some point, the medical community involved in Evelyn's care will determine that curative care is no longer appropriate. That is, the treatments provided to attempt to "cure" Evelyn will likely cause more pain and suffering, rather than a positive outcome. At that point, treatment is usually switched to palliative care. **Palliative care** is aimed at reducing pain and suffering as a person nears the end of his or her life **(Figure 8-1)**. Some patients receive palliative care from their family doctor, while others choose a hospice provider.

When Evelyn and her son speak with the ethics committee, the committee recommends that she move to the hospice wing of the hospital. **Hospice** facilities provide palliative care. Most hospitals have a hospice wing or center. Sometimes, hospice is provided in private centers outside of a hospital setting. Hospice employees will also make home visits or provide guidance at long-term care facilities. Once it is determined that a patient should receive services from a hospice provider,

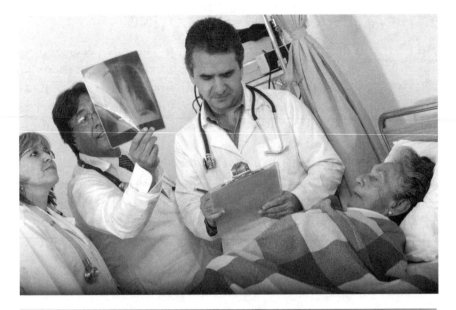

Figure 8-1 Palliative care is for patients whose healthcare providers believe there is no chance of a cure. This type of care is aimed at reducing pain and suffering as a person nears the end of his or her life. Hospice services provide palliative care.

curative care is no longer provided. The only services offered are those that help to alleviate pain and suffering—not prolong life. Evelyn's son argues that her living will states that she wants life support, if necessary. If that is the case, would it not be more appropriate to continue curative treatment?

ADVANCE DIRECTIVES

Advance directives are legally binding statements created by a patient to help that person make wishes known about end-of-life issues **(Figure 8-2)**. There are four types of advance directives: do not resuscitate (DNR) orders, living wills, power of attorney or healthcare proxy designations, and Uniform Anatomical Gift Act, otherwise known as organ donation.

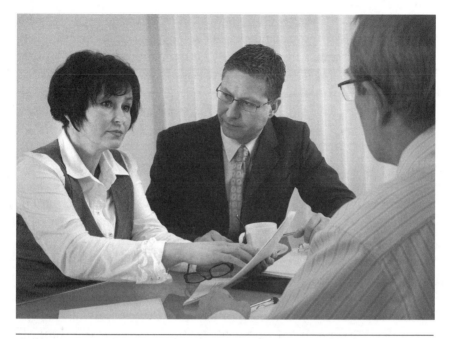

Figure 8-2 Advance directives are legally binding and can be executed by an attorney.

DNR Order

A do not resuscitate (DNR) order informs healthcare professionals that a patient does not want extreme measures taken to save his or her life during cardiac arrest. These measures include cardiopulmonary resuscitation (CPR) and defibrillation. Patients and doctors usually agree to have a DNR order written and placed in the medical record. DNR orders are recommended for patients who have a terminal illness with a prognosis of 6 months or less to live, or who are in the advanced stages of life and would prefer to die naturally. An adult must be competent to request a DNR order. If an adult is not considered competent or is unable to express his or her wishes, a power of attorney or healthcare proxy (described later in this section) might request the DNR order instead.

Ethical complications surrounding DNR orders occur when a patient is brought into the hospital via ambulance and the attending emergency personnel are not aware that the patient has a DNR order in his or her medical chart. Any attempts at resuscitation must be stopped once the DNR order is discovered. To continue with resuscitation efforts would violate a legal document as well as the patient's personal wishes.

Living Will

A **living will** is a legal document that indicates whether a patient wants to be placed on life-prolonging machines (also known as life support) should he or she be unable to communicate personal preferences. Anyone can fill out and place a living will in his or her medical record, but it must be notarized or signed by two witnesses to be considered legal. Regulations on living wills vary from state to state, so it is best to obtain one from a local medical facility or consult a lawyer.

If a patient states in a living will that he or she does not want life support, then the patient cannot legally be placed on any machines. If the patient is placed on life support before the living will is discovered, then the medical team must start the process of withdrawing that life support. *Withdrawing* treatment means discontinuing the treatment once it has already been started. *Withholding* treatment means not starting the treatment because the patient's wishes are known beforehand. It is always legally and ethically easier to withhold life support than to withdraw it. Some healthcare professionals feel that withdrawing life support is against their code of ethics, which is to provide **beneficence**, or promote the well-being of patients. If the patient does not have a living will, a power of attorney or healthcare proxy will need to work with an ethics committee and the attending physician to determine the appropriate course of action. Having a living will provides clear guidelines as to the patient's wishes, which can help prevent controversy.

Included here is an example of a living will. Individuals who plan to use a living will should consult with an attorney first to be sure the information covers all that is necessary and legal to set this type of advance directive in place.

Living Will of

This document is for the purpose of setting forth an advance directive regarding my health and goes to family, healthcare professionals, and any others concerned with my care.

Paragraph AA: I, _____, being of sound mind do willfully and voluntarily record in this writing a pronouncement of procedures to be adhered to concerning my care should I become unable to express or communicate my preferences. I am resolved in my decisions recorded here concerning my right to refuse life-sustaining medical care. I fully expect those listed above (family, doctors, etc.) to abide by these directions and regard them as legally bound to do so. Further, those listed above (family, doctors, etc.) are liability free in following the letter of this living will.

1. I direct my physician(s) to withhold or withdraw life-sustaining care/treatment if its only purpose is to keep me alive.
2. I direct my physician(s) to limit treatment to methods that will keep me as comfortable as possible in my health condition, including those that would stem from withholding or withdrawing life-sustaining care/treatment.
3. I declare that if I am in the condition to need life-sustaining care/treatment, that I specifically DO want the following treatments and/or care:

   a. _____   e. _____
   b. _____   f. _____
   c. _____   g. _____
   d. _____   h. _____

4. I declare that if I am in the condition to need life-sustaining care/treatment, that I specifically DO NOT want the following treatments and/or care:

   a. _____   e. _____
   b. _____   f. _____
   c. _____   g. _____
   d. _____   h. _____

This declaration of my Living Will expresses my unyielding wishes concerning my own health and that I wish to here be executed according to the laws of the State of _____ and still within my own stated wishes.

I make this Living Will Declaration on the _____ day of _____ in the year _____

_____   _____

Signature of Person listed in Paragraph AA
Address of Person listed in Paragraph AA

Case in Point: Terri Schiavo

In the landmark case of Terri Schiavo, the ethical dilemma of withdrawing life support was put on trial. Terri suffered irreversible brain damage due to self-inflicted malnutrition. She was placed on life support and went through several years of therapy. After 15 years, her husband's court-appointed doctors determined that she would most likely not recover and her life support should be discontinued. Terri did not have a living will, so the courts did not have a legal document on which to base a decision. Terri's parents argued that life support and therapy efforts should be continued. The case became a media sensation and resulted in the removal, reinsertion, and then final removal of the feeding tube. An autopsy after her death showed that brain damage was much more severe than they had originally suspected and that recovery would most likely not have occurred. Without a living will, the decision to withdraw life support can be fraught with legal and ethical complications (Schindler v. Schiavo, 2001).

Power of Attorney and Healthcare Proxy

When competent adults are not able to make decisions themselves, they might rely on a power of attorney and/or a healthcare proxy to make decisions for them. A power of attorney is a written document that legally allows someone to make decisions on your behalf. These decisions can be financial or health related. If a separate person is designated to make health decisions on your behalf, they are called a **healthcare proxy** (otherwise known as a **medical power of attorney**). A healthcare proxy designation is not the same as a financial power of attorney, who handles monetary and estate decisions. The same person can be both a financial power of attorney and a healthcare proxy, but some choose to have different individuals handle each role. For example, an elderly widow might designate her son as her financial power of attorney and her daughter as her healthcare proxy. In some instances, financial power of attorneys or healthcare proxies are appointed by the courts. Ethical and legal issues can arise if a patient does not designate these individuals.

Organ Donation

M. Kevin Stump, Chief Executive Officer of the Mississippi Organ Recovery Agency in Jackson, Mississippi, had the following to say about organ donation.

As of March 13, 2012, there are approximately 122,000 people in the United States who are waiting for a lifesaving second chance through an organ transplant. Currently and historically, the list of those waiting continues to grow at a faster pace than donation. To change this, from a preventive standpoint two things must occur: First, we must change lifestyles in the United States to be healthier so that fewer people need transplants. Second, the plague of hepatitis C that we are seeing must be addressed and a solution found. From a donor standpoint, we need to continue to work with the public to ensure their trust in the system and hopefully thereby increase donations. Next, policies that prevent the aggressive transplantation of organs must be lifted, and policies that inhibit organ procurement organizations from placing more organs need to be removed or at least revised.

Ethical policies and procedures must be the cornerstone of the donation and transplantation communities. The system to allocate the scarce organs must be as ethical and fair as possible. Loss of the public's trust in the donation and transplantation system would be devastating to donation rates, and hence more people would die waiting for a second chance.

Courtesy of M. Kevin Stump

Uniform Anatomical Gift Act

The **Uniform Anatomical Gift Act**, passed in 1968, allows anyone 18 years of age or older to donate body parts for the purpose of transplantation after his or her death. It also allows next of kin to give permission regarding the donation of body parts. The law further addresses the donation of bodies for medical research or study. To help simplify and organize the donation of organs, a second law (National Organ Transplant Act) was passed in 1984 (American Organ Transplant Association, n.d.). This act created a network for registering and matching organ donor recipients. The Organ Procurement and Transplantation Network is a private, nonprofit organization that contracts with the federal government.

In an effort to increase the number of organ donations, many states have written laws that allow or require all individuals with a driver's license to designate their organ donor status on their license. This system reduces confusion and can provide clear evidence of a patient's wishes. However, even though most states provide driver's licenses at 16 years of age, an organ donor must have approval from a parent or guardian until 18 years of age.

MAKING END-OF-LIFE DECISIONS

In our case of Evelyn, discussed at the beginning of this chapter, the advance directive she carried was a living will stating that she wanted to be on life support, if necessary. Evelyn's son wanted to discuss curative care options despite the doctor's recommendations of switching to palliative care. While a living will could include such drastic measures, it usually relates to patients who are incapacitated and cannot live without a machine to keep them alive. Evelyn is dying from cancer, but she is able to eat, breathe, and keep her heart pumping without any mechanical intervention. After the ethics committee explains this difference to Evelyn's son, he accepts their recommendation to move Evelyn to the hospice wing of the hospital.

Making decisions regarding end-of-life treatments is difficult. Historically, doctors only provided curative care—often up until the patient requested that treatment stop or simply passed away (Webb, 1999). When life support systems were first introduced, they were seen as a possible new way to keep patients alive indefinitely. One of the first patients to be placed on life support was Karen Ann Quinlan, as discussed in the Case in Point box.

Case in Point: Karen Ann Quinlan

At 21 years of age, Karen Ann Quinlan suffered severe brain damage after a drug and alcohol overdose. She was determined to be in a **persistent vegetative state**, which means that while she appeared to be awake, she did not have enough cognitive function to make voluntary movements and be aware of her surroundings. Karen Ann was placed on life support, which was relatively new technology at the time. After several months, Karen Ann's muscles began to atrophy and it became clear to her family that her quality of life was severely diminished. They requested that she be removed from the ventilator that was keeping her alive. The hospital refused because they were certain that she would die if taken off of the ventilator and they feared litigation from the county prosecutors, who threatened to charge them with homicide. Karen Ann's family took the case to the New Jersey Supreme Court, who ruled in favor of the family. The decision was based on the difference between ordinary and extraordinary means. It was determined that the hospital had an obligation to provide ordinary, but not extraordinary, means and that life support would be considered extraordinary. Interestingly, Karen Ann continued to breathe on her own after the ventilator was removed and finally died of natural causes 9 years later (In re Quinlan, 1976)

About 10 years later, the ethical issue of removing patients from life support would be tested again with the Nancy Cruzan case. When a patient does not have advance directives placed in his or her medical record, it is sometimes difficult for the medical community and next of kin to agree.

Case in Point: Nancy Cruzan

In 1983, Nancy Cruzan was thrown from a vehicle during an accident and landed facedown in a ditch filled with water. She was found without any signs of life, but paramedics managed to revive her. She remained in a coma for several weeks and was finally determined to be in a persistent vegetative state. A feeding tube was inserted for long-term care. Her husband and family waited 7 years for any signs of recovery before deciding it was time to remove all life-sustaining equipment. The hospital argued that Nancy Cruzan was breathing and her heart was pumping without medical intervention, so they would not remove the feeding tube without a court order.

The case went to the Missouri Supreme Court who ruled that clear and convincing evidence of a patient's wishes are needed before a life-sustaining mechanism can be withdrawn. In a conversation before the accident, Nancy had verbally expressed her wishes to not remain alive on life support, but there was no legal document to provide evidence. After the court's decision, the family members were able to gather more proof of Nancy's wishes and eventually the feeding tube was removed. Nancy died 11 days after the feeding tube was removed (Cruzan v. Director, 1990).

The Nancy Cruzan case tested a new issue related to patient rights and state governments. The State of Missouri, as pointed out by the U.S. Supreme Court, places a high importance on the sanctity of life. Other states emphasize the rights of patients to choose their own course of treatment, otherwise known as patient autonomy. This includes the right to choose when their life will end. Two states (Oregon and Washington) have already passed laws allowing terminally ill patients to obtain lethal doses of medication, and several states are considering this option (Euthanasia, n.d.). Oregon was the first state to pass a law related to physician-assisted death.

Euthanasia is a term derived from Greek, meaning "the good death." It refers to the intentional killing of a person to relieve his or her pain and suffering. Some simply refer to the process as "mercy killing."

There are two types of euthanasia: passive and active. **Passive euthanasia** is allowing a patient to die naturally by withholding treatment, including food and water. It is legal in all 50 states and occurs quite often in long-term care facilities when elderly or terminally ill patients start refusing food and water as they near the end of life. Occasionally, it is met with controversy when a patient is on a feeding tube (e.g., the Terri Schiavo and Nancy Cruzan cases) or when a family member requests a feeding tube but the patient's doctor does not recommend one. Research conducted in this area has shown that the insertion of a feeding tube rarely prolongs the life of certain long-term illnesses, such as dementia and Alzheimer's disease (Volicer, 2005).

Physician-assisted death, on the other hand, is considered a form of active euthanasia. **Active euthanasia** is the intentional killing of a patient by non-natural means. Usually it involves a lethal injection of medication, but there are other controversial methods, including depriving patients of oxygen.

Case in Point: Jack Kevorkian

Jack Kevorkian was a doctor and scientist fascinated with the dying process. Starting with a patient who had Alzheimer's disease, Dr. Kevorkian reportedly assisted 130 suicides over the course of 8 years. He invented a machine that allowed patients to self-administer lethal doses of medication in order to end their lives. In an effort to stop his practices, the state of Michigan suspended his medical license and passed a law making assisted suicide illegal. This law was challenged, but the Michigan Supreme Court upheld the law in 1994, stating that assisted suicide was a felony because of common law. (Common law is based on previous court decisions related to the same subject.) They also stated that Michigan's Constitution did not include any protection for suicide assistance. After numerous trials, a Michigan court finally convicted Dr. Kevorkian of second-degree murder in 1999. In this trial, evidence included a videotape that Dr. Kevorkian had sent to the television show *60 Minutes*. In the video, Dr. Kevorkian is shown administering lethal drugs to a patient, which resulted in his death. Dr. Kevorkian was in prison until 2007. His release was contingent on a promise not to assist with any more suicides. He passed away in 2011. Dr. Kevorkian's actions were controversial, and they opened the door for state lawmakers to consider the rights of dying patients (Schneider, 2001).

In 1997, the U.S. Supreme Court recognized that there is no constitutional right to physician-assisted death, but noted that state legislatures could legalize it. This Supreme Court decision gave power to individual states. Oregon was the first state to legalize physician-assisted death when it passed the Death With Dignity Act. This act allows terminally ill patients in Oregon the right to self-administer a lethal dose of medication that is legally prescribed by a doctor. To be eligible, the patients must have a diagnosis of a terminal illness that will cause death within 6 months. The request must be witnessed by two people, and the patient must be free of any mental illness, including depression. Proponents for the law argue for patient autonomy, or the right to make choices regarding treatment, including the method of their death. They also point out that legalizing physician-assisted death helps patients die in a dignified manner without the stigma associated with suicide or loss of life insurance for their survivors. Washington followed suit with similar legislation in 2008, called the Washington Death With Dignity Act. Other state courts are considering the option or have upheld a patient's right to die. For example, in

Baxter vs. Montana (2009), the courts ruled that a patient's right to privacy extends to the decision of terminally ill patients to end their lives with a lethal dose of medication. However, not all states agree. A majority of the states in the United States have existing statutes or common law that prohibits physician-assisted suicide. Any active euthanasia that is not physician assisted is currently illegal in all 50 states.

Healthcare professionals who work in long-term care or hospice facilities are most likely to encounter patients making end-of-life decisions. It is important for all healthcare professionals, however, to consider the ethical implications of advance directives and end-of-life care. When considering treatment options, therapists should know and understand the patient's wishes regarding quality of life. A speech therapist, for example, might be called in to evaluate a patient for feeding tube placement. In addition to evaluating the patient's ability to swallow, the speech therapist should consider the quality of life a patient near the end of life would have with a feeding tube in place. Patients and families should be advised of the pros and cons so they can make appropriate choices. On the clerical side, a medical office manager should be aware of advance directives and where they should be placed in a medical record. They should also make sure those documents are up to date and comply with state laws governing advance directives.

As in our hypothetical case with Evelyn, sometimes an ethics committee can be called in to help make decisions toward the end of a patient's life. These committees examine the options and make recommendations to family members and medical staff. Having clear guidelines, such as advance directives, helps make these decisions easier for all parties.

ETHICAL ISSUES RELATED TO LIFE

After trying to start a family for several years, 43-year-old Abigail and her husband Tony decide to seek fertility counseling. Abigail's good friend is a medical assistant at an OB/GYN office, so she calls on her for advice. Abigail's friend knows that it would be outside of her scope of practice to make any specific suggestions, so she listens politely and recommends that Abigail and her husband make an appointment to see Dr. Reynolds, the OB/GYN in her office. At the appointment, Dr. Reynolds asks several questions, and learning that natural options have not been successful, he recommends considering assisted reproduction.

Assisted reproduction, in general, refers to artificial or semi-artificial methods of achieving pregnancy. Examples include artificial insemination, in vitro fertilization, and surrogacy. During **artificial insemination**, the woman takes drugs to increase egg production, and sperm (from her mate or a donor) is then implanted with a device in an effort to achieve pregnancy. **In vitro fertilization** is one of the most common methods of assisted reproduction. This process involves a woman taking drugs to stimulate egg production. These eggs are collected via a surgical procedure, combined with her mate's sperm (or a sperm donor's), and then reinserted into the uterus. Generally, several eggs are used in the hope that at least one of them will develop into a surviving embryo. While artificial insemination and in vitro fertilization involve having the woman carry the baby herself, **surrogacy** involves having another woman carry the baby from conception to delivery. Assisted reproduction options are most often used by couples who have been unable to conceive or carry a baby to term, or by same-sex couples who wish to have children with a genetic link to one of the parents.

Many ethical issues can arise from assisted reproduction (Asch & Marmor, 2008). Fertility treatments generally come at a high price and are not always covered by insurance policies. This cost reduces the options for couples with limited income who are unable to conceive naturally. In addition, fertility treatments often use a third party—a sperm or egg donor, or even a surrogate mother—who gives up parental rights at the time of donation. During artificial insemination, the sperm donor might request to remain anonymous to avoid an expectation of support in the future. However, the child created from such a union might have a compelling interest to know more about his or her anonymous parent.

In vitro fertilization creates more ethical issues when embryos are created and stored. The embryos that are not used must be kept in storage or destroyed. Pro-life activists (those who argue that life begins at conception, rather than birth) argue that destroying embryos is destroying life. Many scientists would prefer to save unwanted embryos and use them for research. If embryos are created and stored for later use, the issue of how long they can and should be stored is raised. During the in vitro fertilization process, a woman is usually transplanted with several artificially created embryos in an effort to obtain at least one viable pregnancy. This can result in multiple births, usually twins but occasionally triplets or more. Multiple births themselves are not particularly controversial, but they can result in difficult pregnancies, premature births, and/or birth defects. When a multiple birth is created artificially, rather than a natural occurrence, questions about health and welfare can arise. Some would argue that the in vitro fertilization process is an unnecessary procedure that carries potential risk to both the mother and the offspring.

Case in Point: Nadya Suleman

Nadya Suleman gave birth to octuplets in 2009. They were conceived after 12 embryos were implanted during an in vitro fertilization procedure. Nadya reports that only 6 were supposed to be implanted but that during the procedure she was told that the first 6 had been expelled. While carrying octuplets to term is quite controversial, Nadya's situation was even more complicated because she was already a single mother to 6 children. In addition, the implantation of 12 embryos was considered extreme, and as a result the Medical Board of California chose to revoke the license of the doctor involved. All 8 babies were delivered prematurely, and the cost of their hospital stay reportedly cost the taxpayers hundreds of thousands of dollars (Zarembo, 2012).

Surrogacy opens the door to multiple ethical issues as well. Generally, in a surrogate situation, the natural mother is unable to carry a baby to term. In these cases, the egg and sperm come from the natural mother and father, are artificially joined to create an embryo, and are then implanted into the uterus of a surrogate mother. This woman will carry the baby to delivery and relinquish all parental rights at the time of birth. Questions arise as to the amount of contact a surrogate parent can or should have with the child after birth. In the typical 9 months that a baby is carried in utero, a bond is often formed between the carrier and the fetus, making separation difficult at the time of birth. In addition, surrogate mothers earn monetary compensation for their services—usually a fee in addition to medical costs—which some consider unethical because it turns childbirth into a business. Laws regulating surrogacy vary from state to state (Center for American Progress, 2007). Currently, surrogacy contracts are banned in the state of Arizona and in Washington DC. Some states void surrogacy contracts and penalize the people involved in the contract. Other states allow surrogacy, but with restrictions. Before recommending any form of surrogacy, a healthcare professional should consider state laws.

After considering the issues surrounding each option, Abigail and Tony opt for in vitro fertilization. The procedure is successful and Abigail becomes pregnant. An ultrasound shows that she is carrying twins. Abigail and Tony are thrilled and begin to prepare for the arrival of their children. As Abigail's due date nears, she starts to experience some health issues. Dr. Reynolds diagnoses Abigail's condition as preeclampsia—a high blood pressure disorder that affects both the mother and the child during pregnancy. Abigail's condition is quite severe, so she is ordered to bed rest. It appears that Abigail may have to consider an early delivery or risk her own health. After several checkups and no sign of improvement, the nervous couple discusses options with Dr. Reynolds.

Historically, there have been many ethical and legal issues surrounding the rights of an unborn child versus the rights of the mother. As a society, we tend to place a greater emphasis on the rights of the mother, but sometimes the mother will waive those rights in favor of the unborn child or children.

Case in Point: Angela Carder

After several years of battling bone cancer, 27-year-old Angela Carder became pregnant. The cancer had been in remission for 3 years. During the 25th week of pregnancy, a tumor was found in Angela's lung. At the beginning of Angela's pregnancy, she had clearly expressed her wish to have cancer treated if it resurfaced—even at the risk of her fetus. Surgery was not an option, leaving only chemotherapy and radiation in an effort to prolong Angela's life. A decision was made not to induce an early delivery because the infant would be too premature. Angela's health deteriorated, which adversely affected the fetus. The hospital administrator was informed of the situation and expressed concern that only a court order could prevent the delivery of a potentially viable fetus. Although Angela's parents and doctors supported her decision to delay delivery and start treatments to fight the tumor, the hospital required a court order to obey her wishes. Angela was clearly near the end of life but was still able to express her wishes when the court ordered a surgical delivery. The decision was based on the life of a patient dying from cancer versus a potentially viable fetus. Angela verbalized her disagreement with the court, knowing that she would most likely not survive the surgery. The fetus died within 2 hours and Angela Carder died 2 days later. She never received the chemotherapy or radiation treatment requested.

After her death, the Estate of Angela Carder took the issue to the Washington DC Court of Appeals, which ruled that women have a constitutional right to informed consent. This means that medical procedures cannot be completed without consent. They also ruled that the rights of a pregnant mother come before the rights of the fetus (Murphy, n.d.).

In our case of Abigail and Tony, the decision was made to have an early delivery. Both Abigail and Tony agreed that they would rather accept the risks of premature infants than risk Abigail's life. Abigail sat down to talk with her friend, the medical assistant, about their choice. Abigail told her friend that one of the options discussed was abortion—something Abigail never thought she would consider. Abigail's friend admitted that she relied on the conscience clause at her place of work so that she did not have to help with any abortion procedures.

The **conscience clause**, a federal regulatory law, protects health-care professionals from discrimination if they refuse to participate in sterilization procedures or abortions, due to religious or personal objections. The original law included protection for pharmacists and hospitals, but in January 2012, the Obama administration repealed the old law and replaced it with a new one. The new law only protects healthcare professionals who wish to avoid assisting with steriliza-tion and abortion procedures. Opponents of the conscience clause state that healthcare professionals should not be able to opt out of normal job duties simply because they find them offensive. Ethically, it is important for healthcare professionals to research their job duties carefully before accepting a job. Legally, a healthcare professional must tell an employer that he or she wishes to utilize the conscience clause at the time of hire.

Historically, the rights of a mother are placed before the rights of a fetus. This includes the right to have an abortion. An **abortion** is the termination of a pregnancy by removing the fetus from the uterus before it has a chance to become viable. In the landmark case of Roe vs. Wade, the U.S. Supreme Court ruled that a woman's right to privacy extends to fertility decisions. This means that the decision can be made to terminate a pregnancy. In this ruling, the states were given the right to regulate abortion, including placing limitations on when a woman can have an abortion and the need for minors to have parental consent. Many states limit abortions to certain instances, such as when the pregnancy puts the mother's life at risk.

Individuals in favor of abortion usually argue that life does not begin until the time of birth, while individuals against abortion argue that life begins at conception. Studies surrounding fetal development might make these arguments more or less difficult in the future. Another ethical issue that arises in the abortion debate is the rights of the biological father. When the mother wants an abortion but the father does not, or vice versa, who has the superior legal rights? Generally the courts side with the mother, as she is the one who will carry the baby to term. Worldwide, the abortion rate has decreased as access to contraceptives increases. Society, in general, frowns on the use of abortion as a contraceptive.

As a healthcare professional, you may be approached about legal and ethical issues surrounding life. It is important to remember to remain within the appropriate scope of practice and only make recommendations that align with your training and experience.

PUTTING IT ALL TOGETHER

Knowing and understanding the legal and ethical issues surrounding life and death is important in an effort to be a well-rounded healthcare professional. Rather than shying away from controversial topics, it is necessary to understand both sides of an issue in an effort to provide empathetic and compassionate care.

CHAPTER CHECKUP

Matching

A. In vitro fertilization
B. Beneficence
C. Uniform Anatomical Gift Act
D. Advance directive
E. Medical power of attorney
F. Palliative care
G. Abortion

_____1. Aimed at reducing pain and suffering as a person nears the end of his or her life

_____2. Legally binding statement created by a patient

_____3. Promoting the well-being of a patient

_____4. Terminates a pregnancy

_____5. A law that allows people to donate organs

_____6. Another term for healthcare proxy

_____7. A type of assisted reproduction

Discussion

1. In at least one paragraph, discuss one ethical issue about organ donation.
   1. The ability of the patient to pay for treatment and care.
   2. How much the patient's insurance does or does not pay (or if they even have insurance).
   3. Should a person be moved to the top of the organ waiting list if that person's need is the greatest?
   4. Should age be considered in whether or not a person receives an organ?
   5. Should other medical conditions (besides the reason for transplant) be considered in whether or not a person receives an organ?
2. Review the case of Angela Carder in this chapter. Using the three-step model, come to a conclusion about this case.

REFERENCES

American Organ Transplant Association. (n.d.). Uniform Anatomical Gift Act. Retrieved from http://www.a-o-t-a.org/uniform-anatomical-gift-act.html

Asch, A., & Marmor, R. (2008). Assisted reproduction. In _From birth to death and bench to Clinic: The Hastings Center bioethics briefing book for journalists, policymakers, and campaigns (5–10)_. Retrieved from http://www.thehastingscenter.org/Publications/BriefingBook/Detail.aspx?id=2210

Baxter v. Montana. 2009 WL 5155363 (Mont. 2009)

Center for American Progress (2007). _Guide to state surrogacy saws._ Retrieved from http://www.americanprogress.org/issues/2007/12/surrogacy_laws .html/.

Cruzan v. Director, Missouri Dep't of Health, 497 U.S. 261 (1990).

Euthanasia. (n.d.). State laws on assisted suicide. Retrieved from http://euthanasia.procon.org/view.resource.php?resourceID=000132

In re Quinlan, 355 A. 2d 647 (N.J. 1976).

Murphy, J. (n.d.). Angela Carder: A case study in maternal and fetal rights. Retrieved from http://www.nymc.edu/Clubs/quill_and_scope/volume2/murphy.pdf

Schindler v. Schiavo (*In re* Schiavo), 780 So. 2d 176, 180 Fla. Dist. Ct. App. (2001).

Schneider, J. (2001, June 3). Dr. Jack Kevorkian dies at 83; A doctor who helped end lives. Retrieved from http://www.nytimes.com/2011/06/04/us/04kevorkian.html?pagewanted=all

Volicer, L. (2005). End-of-life care for people with dementia in residential care settings. Retrieved from http://www.alz.org/national/documents/endoflifelitreview.pdf

Webb, M. (1999). *The good death: The new American search to reshape the end of life*. New York: Bantam.

Zarembo, A. (2012, January 16). "Octomom" Nadya Suleman's octuplets celebrate 3rd birthday. Retrieved from http://latimesblogs.latimes.com/lanow/2012/01/octomom-octuplets-birthday-nadya-suleman.html

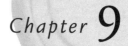

Chapter 9

Controversial Issues in Health Care

Controversial proposals, once accepted, soon become hallowed.

—Dean Acheson

IN THIS CHAPTER, YOU WILL LEARN ABOUT:

- The stem cell research debate
- The ethical implication of genetic testing
- Organ allocation
- The conscience clause—a closer look
- Ethical issues surrounding research

KEY TERMS

Blastocyst

Cloning

Dickey-Wicker Amendment

Deoxyribonucleic acid (DNA)

Eugenics

Genetic testing

Human Genome Project

Stem cells

Sterilization

United Network for Organ Sharing (UNOS)

For Your Consideration

In health care, the bottom line is the health and best interest of the patient. Throughout this text, you have been called upon to reflect on your own value systems; this chapter is no different. You may find it difficult to come to a conclusion on some of these issues, and that is normal. To completely make up your mind, you may need to do some further research in learning all the facts. Knowledge is power.

CONTROVERSY IN HEALTH CARE

Health care involves the health and well-being of individuals. Because people and their needs are complicated, this field will always be surrounded with controversial issues. Many controversial issues make a splash in the media, especially during presidential elections or when scientists discover something new. Most healthcare professionals will not be faced with controversial topics on a daily basis, but a general knowledge of these issues is helpful in understanding our medical world.

THE STEM CELL RESEARCH DEBATE

Stem cells are undifferentiated cells found in embryos that have the ability to self-replicate either as copies of themselves or as copies of other types of cells **(Figure 9-1)**. There are three main sources of

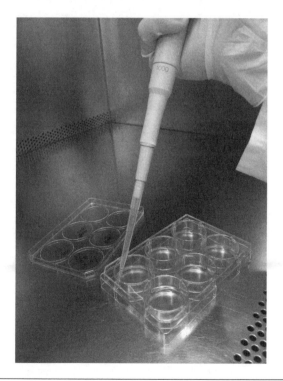

Figure 9-1 Stem cells.

stem cells: bone marrow, umbilical cord blood, and embryos created by in vitro fertilization. Stem cells obtained from bone marrow are known as adult stem cells. Cord blood stem cells are obtained from donated umbilical cords.

Embryonic stem cells are taken from the **blastocyst** that develops shortly after a sperm and an egg are joined together to create a fertilized embryo. While stem cells obtained from cord blood and bone marrow can be taken with the consent of a competent adult, embryonic stem cells involve the destruction of an embryo, which causes controversy.

Scientists involved in stem cell research hope to find cures for diseases and other therapeutic treatments to improve the lives of patients with debilitating injuries and birth defects. Much of the research is experimental, such as a recent case in which doctors used stem cells to regrow blood vessels in a young girl born with a heart defect (Winslow, 2012). Other therapeutic uses for stem cells include treating certain types of childhood leukemia and multiple sclerosis. In the treatment of leukemia, scientists prefer to use stem cells from umbilical cord blood because the cells are more compatible with all body types and appear to grow much more rapidly. Cord blood does not generate a high number of usable stem cells, however, and the donor numbers are generally small. Experimental multiple sclerosis treatment uses stem cells to replace the protective covering of nerve fibers destroyed by the inflicted patient's immune system. It is hoped that a combination of stem cells and other therapies will eventually result in a possible cure for the disease.

If stem cell research appears to have positive outcomes, then why is it considered so controversial? The use of adult stem cells and stem cells obtained from umbilical cords is generally free of controversy. However, as these stem cells are duplicated (for research purposes), they start to lose their effectiveness. In addition, both adult and umbilical cord stem cells have a greater risk of rejection by patients who accept them for therapeutic purposes, as compared to blastocyst stem cells.

Because blastocyst stem cells are created during in vitro fertilization, they are new and therefore have greater potential for therapeutic treatment and less risk for rejection. Taking stem cells from a blastocyst, however, destroys the embryo. This is where the controversy begins (Monroe, Miller, & Tobis, 2007). While these embryos were originally created to help a woman become pregnant, they were never used. These embryos carry the potential for life, but until they are planted in a woman's uterus, they will never become a human being. Does that mean they should be saved indefinitely or discarded, or does the chance to further our scientific knowledge outweigh the potential loss of life? This question is not easily answered, and society might never come to an agreement. Because various religions view the embryo in different lights, it is not likely that a consensus will be reached in the near future **(Table 9-1)**.

While the use of stem cells for research purposes comes with much controversy, another issue surrounding the topic is sources of funding. Even though stem cell research is controversial, there is no federal law prohibiting the research, and most states allow or encourage it. However, both federal and state laws restrict the funding of stem cell research that involves stem cells obtained from embryos.

Table 9-1 Religious Views on the Moral Status of the Embryo and Fetus (Knowles, n.d.)

Religion	View
Roman Catholicism/ Fundamentalist Christianity	Full moral status is obtained at conception; destroying stem cells for research is similar to homicide.
Mainstream Protestantism	Limited moral status is obtained at conception; some Protestant groups support stem cell research, while others do not.
Buddhism and Hinduism	Undecided; conflicted between a mandate to avoid harming other living things and a general support of research that helps others.
Islam	Embryo does not have moral status; supports stem cell research.
Judaism—Orthodox and Conservative	Embryo does not have moral or legal status; supports stem cell research.

An amendment to a federal bill providing funding to the National Institutes of Health prohibits the use of federal funding of research that creates, destroys, or harms embryos. Known as the **Dickey-Wicker Amendment**, it was originally signed in 1995 by President Bill Clinton and has been renewed every year since.

In 2001, President George W. Bush allowed federal funds to be used on stem cell lines already created, but not to create any new lines of stem cells. President Bush felt this was an appropriate compromise because federal funding was being used on stem cell lines created from embryos, but not for the original creation of those embryo lines. In 2009, President Obama reversed President Bush's mandate and allowed federal funding to be used on any stem cells—regardless of how they were originally created. The issue is mostly semantic. The Dickey-Wicker Amendment is written in present tense, which means that federal funding cannot be used to create, destroy, or harm embryos, but it does not prohibit the use of federal funds on stem cells that were created by institutions funded with non-federal money.

The use of federal money to support stem cell research is controversial because taxpayer dollars are being used to support something that society does not necessarily agree is ethical. Some would argue that federal funding should be used to support stem cell research because the presence of federal dollars allows the research findings to fall under federal control instead of into private hands and used for strictly private purposes. This may not be entirely true, though, as even with federal funding, the research outcomes generally belong to the organization that employs the researcher. So, while federal funding itself might come with certain restrictions, it does not necessarily guarantee that therapeutic findings will be shared by all.

The issue of stem cell research and funding is a far way from being settled. It does appear that research will continue—with or without federal funding. As healthcare professionals, there is little we can do to promote or educate on this issue. If patients ask questions or raise concerns, it is always best to refer them to their primary physician. Anything else would be outside the scope of practice of most allied health professionals.

THE ETHICAL IMPLICATIONS OF GENETIC TESTING

In 2003, the **Human Genome Project** succeeded in mapping the human DNA sequence (Human Genome Project Information, 2011). **DNA**, or **deoxyribonucleic acid**, is the small code contained in all human cells that determines our characteristics (Genetics Home Reference, 2012; **Figure 9-2**). While researchers are learning more and more every day about the human DNA sequence, having a map of our personal DNA allows scientists to complete **genetic testing**

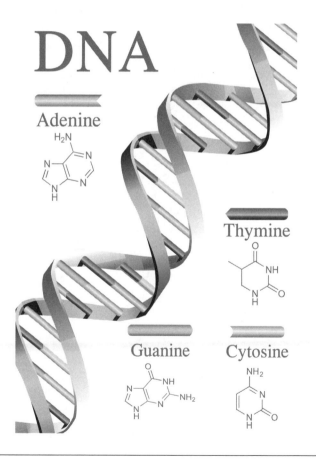

Figure 9-2 DNA strand.

for a variety of purposes. Our legal system uses genetic testing to match samples from crime scenes to criminal suspects. Courts can use genetic testing to establish paternity and thereby ensure that financial support is provided to mothers and their children. In health care, genetic testing can help determine the possibility of developing certain disorders and diseases. While these applications might seem to make genetic testing a fantastic idea, it is full of ethical concerns.

Case in Point: Burlington Northern Santa Fe Railroad

In 2001, Burlington Northern Santa Fe Railroad settled out of court by agreeing to stop secret genetic testing of its employees. The case began after employees filed workers compensation claims for carpal tunnel syndrome (a wrist injury caused by repetitive motion). The company began taking blood samples from other employees and using them to screen for predisposition to carpal tunnel syndrome. (As it turned out, the company was mistaken in thinking the blood test would determine predisposition for carpal tunnel syndrome.) Employees were told the blood testing was mandatory and were not given an explanation. In the out-of-court settlement, no damages were awarded to the employees, but the railroad company did pay the court costs of the unions involved (Philipkoski, 2001).

Genetic testing has a variety of purposes in health care. If a patient has a family history of certain types of cancer, genetic testing might reveal a predisposition for that type of cancer, as well as the potential of passing it along to any biological children. The problem with this type of testing is that it is new and not entirely reliable. Having the predisposition for cancer does not mean a patient will actually develop that cancer. So, if a woman has a family history of breast cancer and genetic testing reveals a predisposition for that type of cancer, should she take preventive measures by having a mastectomy to remove her breasts? This might seem extreme, but to some patients it might seem like a logical step. If individuals do decide to take such preventive treatments, should health insurance companies be required to pay for them, or should they be considered elective, requiring that patients pay for them out of pocket?

Another ethical issue raised by genetic testing is the screening of children for certain traits—either before birth (in utero) or after birth. The Human Genome Project, as well as basic human rights, request that we not reduce individuals to their genetic characteristics, but rather promote the respect of uniqueness and diversity. This does not, however, prevent parents from wanting certain characteristics for their children (e.g., musical or physical ability) or attempting to prevent certain traits or diseases (e.g., diabetes or obesity) **(Figure 9-3)**.

While some researchers consider genetic testing to be a great leap forward, others warn that it might be used for harmful consequences. The misuse of genetic information might seem like something out of a science fiction novel, but in our not-so-distant past, eugenics

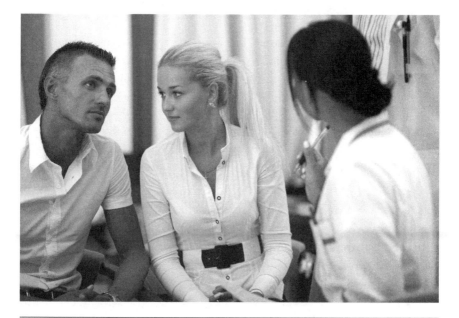

Figure 9-3 Parents sometimes want to have genetic testing done on their unborn child to determine if the child has the potential for any genetic birth defects.

was practiced by certain societies. Known as an effort to improve the genetic makeup of a population, **eugenics** is a very controversial subject. Nazi Germany used this philosophy to justify medical experimentation and even extermination of non-white and Jewish citizens. Even in our own country, certain nonconsenting adults were sterilized in an effort to reduce the risk of continuing the genetic line. For example, certain states passed laws requiring the **sterilization** of patients classified as "mentally ill." These laws were eventually overturned, but not before thousands of patients were sterilized.

Just like stem cell research, it is not likely that genetic testing will disappear in the near future. Rather, it is likely to become more common. As healthcare professionals, it is important to know and understand that patients might have questions and concerns about the potentials of genetic testing. To remain within our scope of practice, these questions should be referred to a patient's primary care giver.

ORGAN ALLOCATION

As discussed previously, one of the advance directives available to patients is the right to donate organs. The Uniform Anatomical Gift Act, passed in 1968, allows anyone 18 years of age or older to donate body parts for the purpose of transplantation after his or her death. It also allows next of kin to give permission regarding the donation of body parts. The law further addresses the donation of bodies for medical research or study. In addition to an advance directive, any living person can volunteer to donate organs.

To help simplify and organize the donation of organs, a second law (National Organ Transplant Act) was passed in 1984. This act created a network for registering and matching organ donor recipients. The Organ Procurement and Transplantation Network (OPTN) is a private, nonprofit organization that contracts with the federal government. Currently, the OPTN is operated by the **United Network for Organ Sharing (UNOS)**. UNOS was awarded the contract in 1986 and focuses on sharing organs from deceased donors in an efficient and equitable manner. They also maintain a waiting list of potential organ recipients and work on educational efforts to increase organ donations nationwide. In response to the shortage of organs available for transplantation, UNOS also raises awareness of live donations, in which living donors give organs to those in need of a transplant (United Network for Organ Sharing, n.d.).

In the United States, the donation of organs has come exclusively from deceased patients or living patients who donate the organs voluntarily without financial benefit. There are significantly more people waiting for donated organs than there are organs available **(Figure 9-4)**. This raises the question of finding new methods of obtaining organs. In some countries donors are paid for organs. Singapore pays donors nearly $36,000 per organ, and Iran has

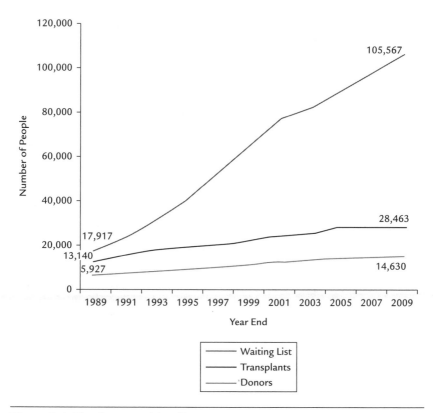

Figure 9-4 The donor–waiting list gap.

eliminated its waiting list for kidney transplants by paying donors. In Israel, if you are not designated as an organ donor, you are placed at the bottom of the recipient list should you need one yourself. Some countries, such as Great Britain, operate under "presumed consent," which allows body parts to be taken at the time of autopsy (Tabarrok, 2010). Most organs are no longer viable by the time an autopsy occurs, but corneas can be used, as well as tissue samples for research purposes.

Interesting Facts About Organ Donation (U.S. Department of Human Services, n.d.)

- The following list shows the percentage of recipients who were still living 5 years after their kidney, heart, liver, or lung transplant, as of May 4, 2009:
    - Kidney: 69.3%
    - Heart: 74.9% **(Figure 9-5)**
    - Liver: 73.8%
    - Lung: 54.4%
- In 2010, 62% of living donors were women. The statistic is reversed for deceased donation.
- In 2010, 67% of all deceased donors were white, 16% black, 13% Hispanic, and 2.3% Asian.
- As of December 2011, the national waiting list was made up of 45% white, 29% black, 18% Hispanic, and 7% Asian.

In the United States, the primary avenue for promoting organ donation has been through marketing, education, and certain state laws requiring citizens to designate their organ donation status on driver's licenses. Ethical issues arise when considering paying for donated organs. For example, would this type of policy prey on lower-income families who might consider selling a kidney to pay off credit card debt? Or would it simply fulfill a need for extra income while meeting the health needs of desperate patients? In addition, if selling organs

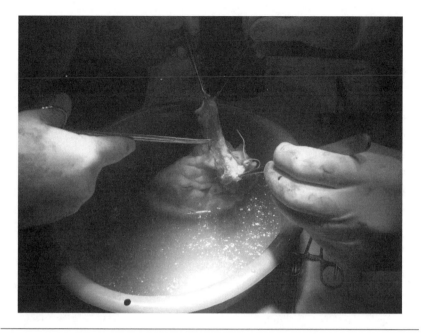

Figure 9-5 Heart transplant.

were to become legal, would regulating quality become too difficult? What if someone were to die because the quality of the organ received was questionable? Recent internet matching services have raised some ethical concerns about informed consent. In these cases, volunteers willingly give an organ to a person who is unfamiliar to them. They are not compensated, except for travel and medical expenses, but some doctors still worry about the ability of the donors to really understand the long-term consequences of their decisions.

When an organ becomes available for transplant, a complex process begins. UNOS maintains a computer database of patients waiting for organ transplantation, and this database is used to find a matching recipient for the donated organ. A variety of factors determine a match, including compatibility, location, and the age and size of both the donor and the recipient. The health condition of both the donor and the recipient is considered as well. Thus, simply being at the top of a waiting list does not guarantee that a patient will receive the next available organ donated.

The effort to match donors and recipients based on these factors leads to some questions about the ethical allocation of donated organs. For example, a large percentage of donated kidneys come from patients of Caucasian descent; yet, nearly a third of patients on the waiting list for kidneys are of African American descent because there is a higher risk of diseases that require kidney transplant in that population. While it is not always necessary to match race for kidney transplantation, there are certain factors that make it easier to match a donor to a recipient from the same race (e.g., similar blood types). Thus, patients of Caucasian descent often wait a shorter time because there is a greater chance of a match being available.

Another issue is health of the patient. Some patients have diminished health after waiting a long time for an organ transplant. This might cause them to drop to a lower transplant status. Is it fair to deny these patients needed organs simply because the long wait has diminished their overall health?

Finally, there is the issue of geographic location. Organs can only survive for a limited time once they are harvested. Therefore, some waiting lists are dependent on proximity to the available organ. Patients with the financial ability to travel on short notice might make arrangements to be on more than one waiting list. For example, Steve Jobs (former CEO of Apple) was able to obtain a liver transplant after placing himself on several waiting lists around the country and using a private plane to jet to the location (Hainer, 2009).

Because of the diversity and large population of our country, the ethical issues surrounding organ donation and allocation are not soon to be resolved. It is not likely that our country will support the buying and selling of organs in the near future, so our current system of donation will continue. As healthcare professionals, we can increase awareness of the need for donated organs and educate patients on the advance directives available to them.

THE CONSCIENCE CLAUSE—A CLOSER LOOK

The conscience clause, a federal regulatory law, protects healthcare professionals from discrimination if they refuse to participate in sterilization procedures or abortions, due to religious or personal objections. The original law included protection for pharmacists and hospitals, but in January 2012, the Obama administration repealed the old law and replaced it with a new one. The new law only protects healthcare professionals who wish to avoid assisting directly with sterilization and abortion procedures.

As discussed previously, one of the ethical dilemmas posed by the conscience clause is whether healthcare professionals should be allowed to decline normal job duties that they find offensive. Healthcare professionals have an ethical obligation to research their job duties carefully before accepting a job. Opponents of this clause pose the question, if a job involves duties to which a person objects, should the person have taken the job in the first place? Legally, a healthcare professional must tell an employer that he or she wishes to utilize the conscience clause at the time of hire.

Case in Point: Catherina Cenzon-DeCarlo

In 2009, Catherina Cenzon-DeCarlo, a devout catholic working as an operating room nurse at Mount Sinai Hospital, was asked to help with an abortion procedure. Ms. Cenzon-DeCarlo had expressed her religious objections to participating in abortion procedures when she interviewed for the job. The abortion was performed on a patient who had preeclampsia—a potentially lethal condition caused by high blood pressure during pregnancy. Ms. Cenzon-DeCarlo alleges that she was led to believe that it was a medical emergency and that the facility did not have time to find a replacement. In addition, supervisors at the hospital threatened to file charges of patient abandonment and insubordination if Ms. Cenzon-DeCarlo did not assist with the procedure. Later, it was determined that the procedure was necessary, but not necessarily an emergency. Ms. Cenzon-DeCarlo filed a lawsuit against the hospital. She still works at the hospital, and the outcome details appear to be confidential (Mucci, 2009).

The Cenzon-DeCarlo case illustrates the importance of healthcare professionals knowing their rights, as well as the ethical issues raised by allowing healthcare professionals to opt out of certain procedures. If this case had truly been an emergency situation, would the outcome of the lawsuit have been different?

Original interpretation of the conscience clause allowed pharmacists to refuse to fill prescriptions used to prevent or terminate pregnancies. State laws have been written to address this issue, as a pharmacist refusing to fill prescriptions raises ethical issues. Some states do not allow pharmacists to refuse to fill prescriptions, while other states allow pharmacists to refuse (National Conference of State Legislatures, 2001). In a healthcare setting, if a nurse refuses to participate in an abortion, a replacement can usually be found. However, in other cases, the solution is not so clear; for instance, if a small town has only one pharmacy, is it fair that patients must obtain medication from another place?

The conscience clause will continue to be tested in the coming years as President Obama's Affordable Health Care Act (AHCA) is challenged in the federal Supreme Court. Currently, the AHCA requires all healthcare policies to provide contraception to patients at low or zero cost. The Catholic Church considers the use of contraception to be a violation of its moral code and therefore does not include it in the healthcare programs available for thousands of individuals who currently work for hospitals and educational facilities owned and run by the Catholic Church.

The Catholic Church does not refuse to allow its employees to use contraceptives. Instead it refuses to pay for the contraceptives as part of a benefits package. The ethical issue at stake is whether or not an employer can force its moral standards on an employee. At the same time, should an employee be able to opt out of job requirements simply because of moral differences?

These are questions that the healthcare community will continue to debate. More detailed policies, as well as state and federal laws, are sure to appear in the years to come. As a healthcare professional, you must be aware of the laws in your state surrounding the conscience clause. If you have moral convictions that might prevent you from participating in certain procedures or from filling certain prescriptions, it is imperative to tell your employer at the time of hire and to be aware of your rights.

ETHICAL ISSUES SURROUNDING RESEARCH

According to the Patient Bill of Rights, patients have the right to decide whether or not to participate in research studies. It is generally agreed that research should always involve informed consent, include only willing and knowing participants, and come at a minimal risk to those involved. There are some gray areas, however, in the research world. For example, very few patients are aware that once a blood or tissue sample is given to a healthcare organization, it becomes the organization's property.

Case in Point: Henrietta Lacks

Henrietta Lacks developed cervical cancer at 30 years of age. Tissue samples of her cancer were taken by a doctor from Johns Hopkins and given to a scientist who was trying to grow lines of human cells to be used for research purposes. Ms. Lacks's cells became the first human cells to grow successfully in an artificial environment, which allowed them to be used to help develop cures for certain diseases, such as polio, as well as to conduct research critical to gene mapping. These cells, named HeLa cells, were used by countless scientists and researchers, who eventually benefitted financially from their research finds. Ms. Lacks's family was unaware that her cells had been used for profit until many years later. Ms. Lacks passed away shortly after her cervical cancer diagnosis, and neither she nor her survivors benefitted financially in any way from this research (Zielinski, 2010).

When patients give blood and tissue samples, they are required to sign consent forms. The question remains, how many patients understand the ethical and legal implications involved? If they do not understand, is it truly informed consent?

Not all healthcare professionals will be involved in research activities. If they are, it is likely that additional training and certification will be required. It is especially important to minimize the risks involved with research including vulnerable populations. Additional laws and ethical principles guide any research involving these populations.

Finally, it is important to note that when experimental treatments are offered to patients for research purposes, it is hard to know if the patient's desire to try a new procedure—any procedure that might cure a disease or alleviate suffering—overshadows the risks. For example, if a patient is in the final stages of cancer and has the option to try an experimental treatment option, is it ethical for a doctor to promote this new procedure or better to offer palliative care? In the end, it is best to provide both options to the patient and let the patient choose what he or she thinks is best.

OTHER CONTROVERSIAL ISSUES

There are many other controversial issues in health care. The issue of cloning is never far off when we discuss stem cell research. **Cloning** is the copying of cells to create copies with similar genetic content. Generally, cloning is considered acceptable for research purposes only (e.g., the cloning of Henrietta Lacks's cells) and will not soon be used for any other purposes. The concept of cloning life forms is considered too controversial at this time. Other controversial issues include abortion, methods of assisted reproduction, and euthanasia.

PUTTING IT ALL TOGETHER

As we continue to learn more about ourselves through research and discovery, there is really no end to the controversies that will arise. The key is to stay educated on these topics so that we can make informed and ethical decisions. Remember—knowledge is power!

CHAPTER CHECKUP

Fill-in-the-Blanks

1. Three common sources of stem cells are _____ _____,
_____ _____ _____, and _____
_____ _____ _____-_____ _____.
2. Scientists involved in stem cell research hope to find _____
for diseases and other therapeutic treatments to _____ the
lives of patients with debilitating injuries and birth defects.
3. In 2003, the _____ _____ _____ succeeded in
mapping out the human DNA sequence.
4. The United Network for Organ Sharing maintains _____
_____ and matches donated _____ to potential
transplant recipients.
5. According to the _____ _____ _____,
patients have the right to decide whether or not to participate in
_____ _____.

True/False

1. All religions disagree with embryonic stem cell research.
2. All funding for stem cell research comes from federal sources.
3. Nazi Germany used the philosophy of eugenics to justify medical
experiments and extermination of citizens.
4. Organs are given out on a first-come, first-served basis.
5. The conscience clause can be used at any time in a healthcare
professional's career.

Discussion

1. Which sources of stem cells are considered less controversial?
2. What do you think is the most fair and equitable method for al-
locating organs?
3. Would you consider genetic testing for yourself or your family?
4. If a patient is considering participating in a research study, what
advice can you give him or her?

REFERENCES

Genetics Home Reference. (2012, March 26). What is DNA. Retrieved from http://ghr.nlm.nih.gov/handbook/basics/dna

Hainer, R. (2009, June 24). Did Steve Jobs' money buy him a faster liver transplant? *CNN.* Retrieved from http://www.cnn.com/2009/HEALTH/06/24/liver.transplant.priority.lists/index.html

Human Genome Project Information. (2011). Retrieved from http://www.ornl.gov/sci/techresources/Human_Genome/home.shtml

Knowles, L. P. (n.d.). Religion and stem cell research. *Stem Cell Network.* Retrieved from http://www.stemcellnetwork.ca/uploads/File/whitepapers/Religion-and-Stem-Cell-Research.pdf

Monroe, K. R., Miller, R., & Tobis, J. (Eds.). (2007). *Fundamentals of the stem cell debate: The scientific, religious, ethical, and political issues.* Berkeley, CA: University of California Press.

Mucci, K. (2009, August 6). Nurse sues hospital after allegedly being forced to assist in abortions. *Health Leaders Media.* Retrieved from http://www.healthleadersmedia.com/page-2/HR-237103/Nurse-Sues-Hospital-After-Allegedly-Being-Forced-to-Assist-in-Abortion

National Conference of State Legislatures. (2001, February). Pharmacist conscience clauses: Laws and information. Retrieved from http://www.ncsl.org/issuesresearch/health/pharmacist-conscience-clauses-laws-and-information.aspx

Philipkoski, K. (2001, April 10). Genetic testing case settled. *Wired.* Retrieved from http://www.wired.com/science/discoveries/news/2001/04/42971

Tabarrok, A. (2010, January 8). The meat market. *The Wall Street Journal.* Retrieved from http://online.wsj.com/article/SB10001424052748703481004574646233272990474.html

United Network for Organ Sharing. (n.d.). Data collection. Retrieved from http://www.unos.org/donation/index.php?topic=data_collection

U.S. Department of Human Services. (n.d.). *Donate the gift of life.* Retrieved from http://www.organdonor.gov/about/data.html

Winslow, R. (2012, March 20). To fix a heart, doctors train girl's body to grow new part. *The Wall Street Journal.* Retrieved from http://online.wsj.com/article/SB10001424052702303812904577291772001385812.html

Zielinski, S. (2010, January 22). Henrietta Lacks' "immortal" cells. *Smithsonian.com.* Retrieved from http://www.smithsonianmag.com/science-nature/Henrietta-Lacks-Immortal-Cells.html

Glossary

Abortion   Removal of the fetus from the uterus before it has a chance of becoming viable, resulting in death.

Acquired immune deficiency syndrome (AIDS)   The final stage for HIV patients. At this point, the body is unable to naturally fight infections, which leaves patients prone to developing illnesses that people with weakened immune systems are not able to fight, such as pneumonia and certain cancers.

Active euthanasia   Intentional killing by unnatural means such as a lethal injection or deprivation of oxygen.

Administrative law   The laws that agencies created by the federal government can implement.

Advance directives   Legally binding medical directions that the patient provides in the event that he or she should become incapacitated or unable to make sound medical decisions.

Age Discrimination in Employment Act of 1967   An act that prohibits employment discrimination against individuals 40 years of age or older.

Americans With Disabilities Act (ADA) of 1992   An act that prohibits discrimination of individuals with physical or mental disabilities.

Applied ethics   A major area of ethics that calls for the investigation of any given debate over a morally based issue. There are two aspects of an applied ethical dilemma: (1) that it is an issue that is controversial (meaning, there are more than one viewpoint on the issue) and (2) that it is clearly classified as a moral issue.

Artificial insemination   A type of assisted reproduction by which the female takes drugs to increase egg production and then sperm is planted (from a donor or her mate) into her uterus to further increase the chance of becoming pregnant.

Assault and battery Historically, assault meant the threat of harm, and battery was the actual physical harm to a person. Currently, most states consider both the threat and the act to come under the single term of assault. This includes unwanted touching.

Assisted reproduction Artificial or semi-artificial means of achieving reproduction. Examples include in vitro fertilization (semi-artificial), artificial insemination (semi-artificial), and surrogacy (artificial).

Assumption of risk The understanding that certain procedures can result in commonly known injuries.

Autonomy A person's ability to make decisions concerning his or her own well-being, including health care.

Beneficence The act of doing good and/or showing care for others.

Blastocyst A structure in early fetal development containing a variety of cells from which an embryo develops.

Borrowed servant rule A legal defense generally used by employers who have temporary workers or medical professionals who fill in for other medical professionals on leave. If a plaintiff sues a healthcare facility regarding the actions of an employee on temporary employment, the facility might utilize the borrowed servant rule and escape liability for injury caused by the temporary employee.

Breach To violate.

Breach of duty The failure of a healthcare professional to act as any ordinary and prudent healthcare professional within the same community would act in similar circumstances. There are three categories of breach of duty: misfeasance, malfeasance, and nonfeasance.

Causation The cause. It requires the injury to be closely related to the healthcare professional's negligence.

Child abuse Harm of a person younger than 18 years of age, including physical, sexual, or emotional mistreatment, or neglect.

Civil action A type of statutory law that is considered to be a wrong between individuals, such as defamation of character.

Civil Rights Act of 1964 An act that prohibits the discrimination of anyone based on sex and race during the hiring, promoting, and firing processes.

Cloning The scientific copying of cells to create copies with similar genetic content.

Common law Established by the outcome of court cases.

Comparative negligence A type of negligence in which the plaintiff's actions helped cause the injury. The difference between this type and contributory negligence is that the plaintiff can recover damages based on the amount of the defendant's fault.

Competent Able to make decisions necessary to live independently.

Confidentiality In health care, the duty of keeping personal medical information private.

Conscience clause A federal regulatory law that protects the healthcare professional who refuses to assist in fertilization procedures, including abortion, due to religious or personal objections.

Consent A patient's expression of agreement to treatment.

Consequence The result of an action.

Consequential approach An approach to ethics by which issues are judged as intrinsically (from within) good or bad and the result of an action is based on the decision that will bring about the best balance of good outcomes over bad.

Consolidated Omnibus Budget Reconciliation Act of 1985 (COBRA) A forerunner to HIPAA, legislation that requires businesses with 20 employees or more to provide to employees who leave that business extended health insurance for up to 18 months. This can be at the expense of the company but usually is paid for by the employee.

Constitutional law All laws must be upheld by the U.S. Constitution and any new law written must comply with the Constitution.

Contract for care An agreement that creates a relationship wherein the healthcare provider is to provide care to the patient.

Contributory negligence A type of negligence that occurs when the patient or others are determined to be fully or in part responsible for the injury. In this case, the plaintiff is not able to receive monetary compensation for damages.

Countertransference   The instance of a provider experiencing feelings for a patient that are out of the norm, such as love, anger, or any other emotion.

Criminal action   A violation of statutory law that is considered a wrong against society, such as murder.

Curative care   Care that is used to resolve a patient's condition.

Damages   Injuries caused by the defendant for which compensation is due.

Defamation of character   Damage that is caused to a person's reputation through spreading untrue information, whether by spoken (slander) or written (libel) word.

Denial   The most commonly used defense in cases of negligence. The defendant does not claim that damages did not occur, but rather that there was another explanation or cause for the damages.

Deontology   An approach to ethical dilemmas that maintains that certain life obligations should be of primary focus in a person's everyday life. Those obligations should take priority over others. Also known as rights-based ethics or duty-based ethics.

Deoxyribonucleic acid (DNA)   The small code contained in all human cells that determines each person's characteristics.

Dickey-Wicker Amendment   An amendment to a federal bill providing funding to the National Institutes of Health that prohibits the federal funding of research that creates, destroys, or harms embryos. Signed in 1995 by President Bill Clinton, it has been renewed every year since.

Dignity   The sense of having been treated with respect.

Dilemma   A crisis or situation where a decision is required in order for improvement to occur.

Do not resuscitate (DNR) order   A type of advance directive indicating that no extreme measures are to be taken should the patient go into cardiac arrest.

Doctrine of *res ipsa loquitur*   A Latin expression for "the thing speaks for itself." If the negligent act is so obvious that it appears there could be no other responsible party, the burden of proof shifts to the defendant to prove that he or she is not responsible for the injury. Common examples in health care include amputation of the wrong limb or sponges left in the body after surgery.

Doctrine of *respondeat superior*   A Latin expression for "let the master answer," meaning that employers are responsible for their employees' actions.

Domestic abuse   The willful intimidation, assault, or other abusive behavior committed by one family member or intimate partner against another. These types of cases are often difficult to confirm, but if a healthcare professional suspects that a patient is involved in a domestic abuse situation, it should be reported to the proper authorities.

Duty   A healthcare professional's obligation to treat a patient.

Duty-based ethics   An approach to ethical dilemmas that maintains that certain life obligations should be of primary focus in a person's everyday life. Those obligations should take priority over others. Also known as rights-based ethics or deontology.

Elder ebuse   Any harmful treatment of an elderly person, including physical, emotional, or sexual abuse; neglect; financial exploitation; and self-abuse.

Electronic medical record (EMR)   A medical record that is documented on and available by computer.

Embezzlement   The conversion to your own use of property that you can rightly access but do not own. Embezzlement is not the same as stealing because in cases of embezzlement, the employee has legal access to the funds, but chooses to take some for their personal use.

Empathy   In health care, the quality of treating patients as you would wish to be treated and understanding patient needs.

Equal Employment Opportunity Commission (EEOC)   An agency that oversees several laws, such as the Equal Pay Act, to ensure that discrimination is not used in hiring practices.

Equal Pay Act   An act that prohibits sex-based wage differences between men and women employed in the same establishment who perform jobs that require equal skill, effort, and responsibility and that are performed under similar working conditions.

Ethics   A branch of philosophy concerned with moral considerations.

Eugenics   A controversial science that advocates the use of practices geared toward improving the genetic composition of a population. Adolph Hitler used eugenics during World War II.

Euthanasia   The intentional killing of another person to relieve pain and suffering. In Greek, it means "the good death." There are two types of euthanasia: active and passive.

Fair Labor Standards Act of 1938 (FLSA)   Legislation that sets minimum wage limits, regulates overtime pay standards, and establishes guidelines for youth employment. All employers must comply with the FLSA, except small independently owned construction, retail, and service businesses.

False imprisonment   The holding of a patient against his or her will. This includes the use of restraints for nonmedically approved reasons.

Family and Medical Leave Act (FMLA)   An act that requires employers, given qualifying circumstances, to allow employees up to 12 weeks of unpaid job-protected leave each year after at least 1 year of employment that includes at least 1,250 hours of employment.

Fidelity   In the field of ethics, loyalty.

FLOAT   An acronym for the preferred characteristics of a medical record: **F**actual, **L**egible, **O**bjective , **A**ccurate, and **T**imely.

Fraud   A deceitful practice that deprives someone of his or her rights. An example of fraud in the healthcare field would be making promises to a patient that cannot be kept (i.e., promising the patient that he or she will get better).

Genetic tests   Tests that can determine specific traits in humans. In health care, genetic testing offers a variety of tests to determine the possibility of developing certain disorders and diseases.

Good Samaritan law   A law that protects the healthcare provider from being sued when performing medical care in good faith.

Guardian ad litem   A person who acts as the legal guardian for all decision-making processes, including decisions regarding health care.

Health Insurance Portability and Accountability Act of 1996 (HIPAA)   An act that addresses privacy issues and continuation of health insurance coverage in health care.

Healthcare consumer   Anyone seeking professional care or treatment for health.

Healthcare Integrity and Protection Data Bank (HIPDB)   A national data bank established under HIPAA to prevent fraudulent and/or abusive healthcare practitioners and suppliers from being able to practice. It became fully operational in 2000.

Healthcare proxy   A type of advance directive that assigns a person to make medical decisions for another person. The patient must personally designate the other person. Also known as medical power of attorney.

HELP model   An approach recommended when working with culturally diverse populations: **H**ear what the patient perceives to be the problem; **E**ncourage the patient and healthcare professional to discuss the similarities and differences; **L**ist treatment options and make recommendations; and **P**rovide a chance to negotiate treatment

Hopper   A patient who switches from doctor to doctor.

Hospice   A service that provides palliative care.

Human Genome Project   An effort that succeeded in mapping out the human DNA sequence.

Human immunodeficiency virus (HIV)   A virus that attacks cells in the body that are responsible for fighting infection and disease. Over time, the HIV virus may lead to AIDS.

Implied consent   Consent that occurs when a patient's behavior suggests compliance.

In vitro fertilization   A type of assisted reproduction to stimulate egg production. The eggs from the female are collected through a surgical procedure, combined with sperm (mate's or donor's), then reinserted into the uterus.

Inductive reasoning   Critical thinking that moves from specific details to generalities.

Informed consent   Consent that occurs when the physician explains the treatment or procedure and the patient or patient representative agrees to have it performed. The consent can be verbal, but it is usually written.

Intentional tort   Wrongdoing that is done with malice or forethought.

Invasion of privacy   In the healthcare field, the intrusion into the private life of another person without medical cause. This is different than a violation of HIPAA's Privacy Rule because invasion of privacy extends farther than protected health information. Any damaging information that is made public regarding any employee or patient in a healthcare setting can be considered invasion of privacy.

Liability insurance   Financial protection from claims that arise from patients who are harmed while under the care of a healthcare professional. Most healthcare providers need to buy some form of professional liability insurance.

Living will   A legal document and a type of advance directive that instructs whether the patient wants to be placed on life-prolonging machines (also known as life support) should he or she be unable to communicate personal preferences.

Malfeasance   Negligence with mal-intent (e.g., holding a noncooperative patient too tightly when drawing blood, which results in bruising).

Mandatory reporting laws   Laws requiring healthcare professionals to report suspected cases of abuse. These laws vary from state to state, but in general anyone involved in education, health care, or social work must complete training sessions regarding mandatory reporting.

Mature minor doctrine   A doctrine that provides greater autonomy to minors older than 16 years of age who understand and consent to relatively simple medical procedures. This doctrine is a legal concept used by the courts, but a few states have passed it as a statute.

Medicaid   A federally sponsored program providing assistance to low-income individuals and families to pay the cost of health care.

Medical power of attorney A type of advance directive that assigns a person to make medical decisions for another person. The patient must personally designate the other person. Also known as healthcare proxy.

Medical practice acts Laws that govern licensure and certification in the medical field. They vary from state to state.

Medical record A written story of a patient's medical history. It includes personal information such as name, address, and insurance details. It also includes medical information based on patient visits and other contacts with the patient.

Medicare A federally sponsored program providing healthcare coverage for adults 65 years of age and older, as well as some adults younger than 65 years of age with certain disabilities. It is divided into Parts A, B, C, and D.

Meta-ethics The branch of ethics concerned with the nature of ethics and the source. The *ethics of ethics.*

Misfeasance A wrongdoing that occurs when a mistake is made (e.g., giving the patient the wrong medication).

Negligence In health care, failure of the healthcare professional to uphold an appropriate standard of care. There are four requirements in determining negligence: duty, breach of duty, causation, and damages. Also referred to as unintentional tort.

Noncompliance Failure of a patient to follow a doctor's advice.

Nonfeasance Failure to act (e.g., forgetting to turn a patient, which results in bed sores).

Normative ethics Standards by which right and wrong are determined within a society, often referred to as "the norm." The Golden Rule is an example of normative standards.

Occupational Safety and Health Act Legislation administered by the Occupational Safety and Health Administration (OSHA) that regulates the safety and health conditions of most private and public work environments.

Palliative care Care for the patient that is aimed at reducing pain and suffering toward the end of life.

Passive euthanasia   The act of allowing a person to die by withholding treatment and nourishment (food and water).

Patient Care Partnership   A document, often in brochure form, developed by the American Hospital Association that is given to patients to let them know their rights and responsibilities. It replaced the Patient's Bill of Rights.

Patient Protection and Affordable Care Act   An act that includes the requirement that employees provide reasonable break time for new mothers to pump breast milk.

Patient Safety and Quality Improvement Act   Legislation, published in 2005 and effective in 2009, that launched a reporting system for violations of patient safety.

Patient's Bill of Rights (PBOR)   An important piece of consumer protection, developed in 1973 with a revision in 1992, that seeks to protect the rights of the U.S. patient. It has recently been replaced by the Patient Care Partnership. Both documents were developed by the American Hospital Association.

Persistent vegetative state   A condition in which the patient may appear to be awake but lacks cognitive functioning to make voluntary movements and be aware of his or her surroundings.

Personal values system   A set of beliefs held by an individual.

Portability   A guarantee that there will be no lapse of healthcare coverage when a person changes from one job to another, even when insurance carriers change.

Power of attorney (POA)   A written document that legally allows someone to make decisions on another's behalf. There are several different types of POAs, including, but not limited to, healthcare proxy, healthcare agent, healthcare surrogate, and power of attorney for health care. The terms and definitions vary from state to state.

Preexisting condition   An ailment or disease that the patient already has before health insurance coverage begins.

Pregnancy Discrimination Act of 1978   An act that makes it illegal for an employer to refuse to hire a woman who is pregnant.

Privacy Act of 1974   An act that addresses a variety of private information, including how social security numbers can be shared. It is not exclusive to medical information. The Privacy Act only applies to U.S. citizens and permanent residents, so only those individuals may sue under the statutes of the act.

Privacy Rule Effective in 2001 and fully implemented in 2003, the portion of HIPAA that refers to personal data (past, present, and future), otherwise known as protected health information (PHI).

Progressive discipline model An approach that encourages the employee to improve job performance, rather than receive disciplinary actions from the employer. These types of models vary but typically involve the following steps: (1) Provide counseling or a verbal warning; (2) give a written warning with specific guidelines for improved performance; (3) suspend or demote the employee; and (4) terminate the employee.

Protected health information (PHI) Personal data (past, present, and future). PHI is specific medical information of the patient, such as name, date of birth, or social security number.

PYTHON principle An easy way to posture yourself for prevention of legal action in health care: **P**rotect **Y**ourself; **T**hink **H**onestly; **O**bserve **N**aturally.

Rehabilitation Act of 1973 An act that prohibits employers from discriminating against qualified individuals based on disability. This means that if a disabled individual is able to perform the job duties required with minimal accommodations from the employer, he or she is protected from discrimination.

Release of information A document that allows the healthcare provider to share certain information (not necessarily the whole record).

Respect The act of showing a person attention and regarding the person's feelings.

Rights-based ethics An approach to ethical dilemmas that maintains that certain life obligations should be of primary focus in a person's everyday life. Those obligations should take priority over others. Also known as duty-based ethics or deontology.

Ryan White HIV/AIDS Program A federal program administered by the Health Resources and Services Administration that focuses on providing funding for health care and support services to patients with HIV/AIDS.

SOAP charting method   An approach often used to make for a more consistent record. SOAP stands for **S**ubjective, **O**bjective, **A**ssessment, and **P**lan of action. By using this method, entries are easy to track throughout the record by category and, therefore, may even save time for the physician(s) reviewing it.

Scope of practice   The roles and responsibilities of a professional to which he or she should adhere. A professional should not overstep professional boundaries to do the work of another professional for which he or she is not trained.

Standard of care   The attention given to a task (with a patient) that would be reasonably expected of anyone in a similar situation.

Statute of limitations   A policy that determines how long a plaintiff has to file a claim of negligence. In medical malpractice cases, the statute of limitations begins at the time the injury is discovered. States have their own statutes of limitations, but in general they are 3 to 7 years.

Statutory law   Laws created by the federal and state governments that start as bills, are approved by both legislative branches (Senate and House of Representatives), and eventually are signed by the president (federal laws) or governor (state laws). All statutory laws and executive orders must comply with the Constitution.

Stem cells   Undifferentiated cells found in embryos that have the ability to self-replicate either as copies of themselves or as copies of other types of cells. There are three main sources of stem cells: bone marrow, umbilical cord blood, and embryos created by in vitro fertilization.

Sterilization   A procedure that disables a human from reproducing.

Subpoena duces tecum   A Latin expression for "bring with you under penalty of punishment." In health care, it means send only the portion of information (such as with a medical record) requested.

Surrogacy   A type of assisted reproduction in which another woman carries the baby from conception to birth, then gives the baby to the designated parents.

The Joint Commission (TJC) A federal accreditation agency that reviews patient documentation. It is a not-for-profit agency and was established in 1951.

Three-Step Ethical Decision-Making Model A decision-making model that calls on the decision maker to ask the following: (1) Is it legal? (2) Is it balanced? (3) How does it make me feel?

Title X A federal family planning program.

Tort A Wrong-doing against an individual. It is a type of statutory law.

Transference The instance of a patient transferring feelings or attitudes retained from childhood onto the healthcare provider.

Uniform Anatomical Gift Act Federal legislation passed in 1968 that allows people 18 years of age or older to donate his or her own body parts for use in transplantations after he or she dies. This is a type of advance directive.

Unintentional tort See *negligence*.

United Network for Organ Sharing (UNOS) An agency that operates and oversees the Organ Procurement and Transplantation Network (OPTN). It is a private, nonprofit organization that contracts with the federal government. UNOS also maintains a waiting list of potential organ recipients and works on educational efforts to increase organ donations nationwide.

Utilitarian-based ethics An approach to ethical dilemmas that suggests that decisions should be based on the choice that is best for the majority.

Virtue-based ethics An approach to ethics that encourages the most admirable of virtues within a person's character. Examples include honesty, courage, and perseverance.

Withholding or withdrawing medical treatment Withdrawing treatment means discontinuing the treatment once it has already been started. Withholding treatment means not starting the treatment because the patient's wishes are known beforehand.

Index

Photo Credits

Chapter 1
Opener © JustASC/ShutterStock, Inc.; **1-1** © Andrew Gentry/ShutterStock, Inc.; **1-2** © Philip Lange/ShutterStock, Inc.; **1-3** © Georgios Kollidas/ShutterStock, Inc.; **1-5** Courtesy of Library of Congress Prints and Photographs Division Washington, D.C. 20540 USA

Chapter 2
Opener © Alexander Raths/ShutterStock, Inc.

Chapter 3
Opener © dundanim/ShutterStock, Inc.; **3-1** © Zurijeta/ShutterStock, Inc.; **3-2** © Yuri Arcurs/ShutterStock, Inc.; **3-3** © Claudio Rossol/ShutterStock, Inc.; **3-4A** © StockLite/ShutterStock, Inc.; **3-4B** © Monkey Business Images/ShutterStock, Inc.; **3-4C** © Kurhan/ShutterStock, Inc.; **3-4D** © Blaj Gabriel/ShutterStock, Inc.; **3-5** © Phase4Photography/ShutterStock, Inc.

Chapter 4
Opener © FreshPaint/ShutterStock, Inc.; **4-1** Courtesy National Library of Medicine; **4-2** © Lisa F. Young/ShutterStock, Inc.; **4-3** © auremar/ShutterStock, Inc.; **4-4** © Aspen Photo/ShutterStock, Inc.; **4-5** © wavebreakmedia ltd/ShutterStock, Inc.; **4-6** © Alexander Raths/ShutterStock, Inc.

Chapter 5
Opener © Sergej Khakimullin/ShutterStock, Inc.; **5-1** © Alexey Stiop/ShutterStock, Inc.; **5-2** © Bondarenko/ShutterStock, Inc.

Chapter 6
Opener © SNEHIT/ShutterStock, Inc.

Chapter 7
Opener © Glam/ShutterStock, Inc.; **7-2** © Goodluz/ShutterStock, Inc.; **7-3** © alexskopje/ShutterStock, Inc.

Chapter 8
Opener © ZF/ShutterStock, Inc.; **8-1** © Andresr/ShutterStock, Inc.; **8-2** © Alexander Raths/ShutterStock, Inc.

Chapter 9
Opener © Sebastian Kaulitzki/ShutterStock, Inc.; **9-1** © Jens Goepfert/ShutterStock, Inc.; **9-2** © Webspark/ShutterStock, Inc.; **9-3** © Vadym Drobot/ShutterStock, Inc.; **9-4** © kalewa/ShutterStock, Inc.; **9-5** © kalewa/ShutterStock, Inc.